STEVE JAY

Omicron Unveiled: Navigating the New Normal"

Contents

Introduction

Setting the Stage: The Emergence of the Omicron Variant

In the quiet hum of a world already accustomed to the unsettling cadence of a pandemic, the arrival of Omicron sent ripples through the fabric of our collective existence. It was not just another wave; it was a seismic shift that caught even the most seasoned observers off guard. As the news headlines flashed, and whispers of a new variant spread like wildfire, a global sigh of frustration and trepidation echoed across continents.

In the heart of bustling cities and the serene corners of rural landscapes, people found themselves at the intersection of anxiety and uncertainty once more. The Omicron variant, a name that seemed to materialize from the pages of a dystopian novel, swiftly became the protagonist in a real-life drama none of us had auditioned for.

The journey of Omicron's emergence unfolded against the backdrop of a world we thought we knew, albeit one forever altered by the preceding chapters of the COVID-19 saga. The virus, which had become an unwelcome lodger in our lives, took an unexpected turn. Omicron emerged as a testament to the virus's uncanny ability to evolve, presenting a plot twist in a narrative that was already fraught with twists and turns.

As scientists peered into their microscopes and policymakers grappled with unfolding data, the human experience of this new chapter played out in homes, hospitals, and streets. Fear lingered in the air, mingling with the scent of sanitizer and the taste of uncertainty. The Omicron variant was not merely a scientific anomaly; it was a force reshaping the contours of our reality.

From the moment the first reports trickled in, society found itself thrust into a new act of a drama that seemed to have no final curtain. The variant's arrival challenged the resilience we had cultivated during the previous phases of the pandemic. It was as if nature, in its enigmatic way, had decided to test the limits of our adaptability and strength.

The initial days were marked by a sense of déjà vu—a bitter reminder of the times when the world collectively held its breath, waiting for a new chapter to unfold. The virus, ever the unpredictable storyteller, wove a tale of mutation that transcended borders and blurred the lines between nations. As Omicron crossed continents, it brought with it a renewed sense of vulnerability, a reminder that our interconnected world is both a source of strength and a conduit for unseen threats.

The narrative was not confined to laboratories and research papers. It spilled onto the streets, where conversations shifted from daily routines to the latest updates on Omicron. Faces masked not just against the virus but also against the uncertainties that loomed in the air. Supermarkets, once scenes of panic buying during earlier waves, again witnessed the quiet shuffling of feet as individuals stocked up on essentials, silently preparing for an indeterminate period of disruption.

In the age of instant information, the emergence of Omicron was not just a biological event; it was a social media spectacle. Tweets and posts became the modern-day town criers, disseminating news, opinions, and a myriad of emotions. The virtual world, a refuge for many during lockdowns, transformed into an arena of speculation and concern.

The sense of urgency was palpable, but so was the weariness. The fatigue of endless adaptations weighed on shoulders already burdened by the struggles of the past. It was a moment that tested not only our scientific acumen but also our emotional fortitude. How much more could a world, already stretched thin, endure?

Significance of Understanding and Navigating the New Normal

As the Omicron variant took center stage, it became abundantly clear that we were not merely witnesses to a biological phenomenon; we were active participants in the unfolding narrative. Understanding the significance of this new normal became paramount, transcending the realm of science to touch the core of our shared humanity.

The new normal was not just a catchphrase but a dynamic state of being, a continual negotiation between the familiar and the unknown. It beckoned us to reassess our assumptions, challenge our resilience, and reimagine the very essence of what it means to be human in the face of an invisible adversary.

In navigating this uncharted territory, the need for collective understanding became evident. The significance of comprehending not just the scientific intricacies of the variant but also its societal and cultural ramifications underscored the gravity of the moment. We were not confronting a mere biological entity; we were grappling with a catalyst for profound shifts in the way we live, connect, and envision the future.

The new normal demanded more than passive acceptance; it required active engagement. It beckoned us to sift through the noise of information overload and discern the narratives that truly mattered. It called for a collective introspection on the values that would guide us through the uncertainty, urging us to find common ground in the midst of diversity.

As we delved into the complexities of this evolving reality, it became apparent that the Omicron variant was not just a disruptor; it was a mirror reflecting the strengths and vulnerabilities of our global society. Navigating the new normal meant confronting our fears, embracing our shared humanity, and envisioning a future shaped not only by the challenges we faced but by the resilience with which we faced them.

In the chapters that follow, we will embark on a journey through the intricacies of the Omicron era, exploring the societal and cultural shifts that reverberate through our daily lives. Each chapter will unravel a layer of this complex narrative, inviting readers to navigate the uncharted waters of the new normal with a deeper understanding of the world that emerged from the shadows of the Omicron variant.

The Arrival of Omicron

Tracing the Initial Reports and Global Response

The story of Omicron's arrival unfolded like a suspenseful novel, with whispers of a new variant gradually crescendoing into a global chorus of concern. The initial reports, much like the virus itself, were elusive, surfacing in fragments and leaving the world to piece together a narrative that would reshape the course of the ongoing pandemic.

It began, as many stories do, in the quiet corridors of laboratories and research institutions, where scientists meticulously monitored the genetic makeup of the virus. In the midst of routine surveillance, a sequence of nucleotides caught the discerning eyes of researchers—a code that hinted at a deviation from the known script of the virus. The discovery sent a ripple through the scientific community, a subtle tremor that hinted at the possibility of a new chapter in the pandemic narrative.

As researchers scrambled to understand the implications of this genetic anomaly, the first reports emerged cautiously, almost hesitantly, in scientific journals and forums. The name "Omicron" made its debut, not as a harbinger of doom but as a label for a variant that demanded scrutiny. Initial reports were laden with scientific jargon, describing mutations and genetic markers that only a handful could decipher. The language of the laboratory, however, was soon translated into the lingua franca of global awareness.

News outlets picked up the scent, and the first headlines whispered of a new variant on the horizon. The world, already wearied by the ebb and flow of pandemic news, greeted the reports with a mix of resignation and curiosity. The term "Omicron" soon transcended scientific circles, finding its way into conversations at dinner tables and watercoolers. It became a protagonist in the global narrative, a character that everyone knew by name but few understood.

In the early days, ambiguity shrouded Omicron. Was it more transmissible? Did it pose a greater risk of severe illness? The questions echoed through the uncertainty, and the void was filled not just by scientists but by a cacophony of voices on social media and news platforms. The initial reports, like seeds planted in fertile soil, sprouted a forest of speculation, each tree bearing the fruit of a different narrative.

Governments, caught between the imperative to share information and the fear of inducing panic, navigated the delicate balance of public communication. Press conferences became theaters of reassurance and caution, with leaders attempting to distill complex scientific findings into digestible soundbites. The global response, initially characterized by a measured alertness, soon tiptoed into the terrain of heightened vigilance.

Borders became both barriers and bridges in the face of Omicron's arrival. Nations, scarred by the memories of earlier waves, hesitated to throw open their gates. Travel restrictions, once the exception, now became the rule. Airports, once bustling hubs of connection, transformed into arenas of precaution, where masks and tests became the passport stamps of an era defined by a microscopic adversary.

The global response was not uniform; it mirrored the diversity of the world it sought to protect. Some nations, scarred by the experiences of previous variants, swiftly closed ranks, tightening restrictions and bolstering defenses. Others, perhaps influenced by a sense of fatigue or the belief in the inevitability of viral spread, approached the news with a mixture of caution and pragmatism.

In the heart of this global symphony of responses, the scientific community played a pivotal role. Collaborations that transcended borders became the norm, with researchers sharing data and insights at an unprecedented pace. The collective gaze of scientists turned toward Omicron, attempting to decipher its behavior and predict its trajectory. The race against time had a new competitor, and laboratories worldwide became battlegrounds where the weapons were not chemicals but knowledge.

As the initial reports disseminated and the global response unfolded, the human drama of Omicron's arrival became a tale of shared vulnerability and resilience. It was a reminder that, in the face of an invisible adversary, our interconnected world required not just scientific acumen but a collective spirit of cooperation and understanding.

Public Perceptions and Concerns

In the theater of public perception, Omicron was not just a scientific curiosity; it was a living, breathing entity that stirred the waters of collective consciousness. The whispers of a new variant permeated everyday conversations, seeping into the spaces where hopes and fears collided.

Public perceptions of Omicron were shaped by a myriad of factors—previous experiences with the pandemic, trust in authorities, and the omnipresent influence of social media. The uncertainty surrounding the variant became fertile ground for the growth of speculation, and narratives, both grounded in scientific understanding and unfounded in reality, blossomed in the minds of individuals around the globe.

The first wave of public concern was like a ripple that expanded from the epicenter of scientific discourse to the farthest corners of society. As headlines blared and notifications buzzed, a collective gaze turned toward the latest protagonist in the COVID-19 saga. Social media, the modern-day agora, became a battleground of narratives, where information and misinformation engaged in a relentless dance.

In this landscape of digital discourse, public reactions were as diverse as the global tapestry itself. Some individuals, seasoned by the experiences of earlier waves, approached the news with a stoic resolve, adapting their behaviors with a familiarity born of necessity. For others, the arrival of Omicron reignited the embers of fear, stoking concerns about the unknown and the potential for another upheaval in their lives.

Trust, a fragile currency in the realm of public health, played a pivotal role in shaping perceptions. Those who had weathered the storm of previous waves with confidence in the guidance of health authorities continued to anchor their beliefs in science. For others, skepticism lingered, fueled by the echo chambers of online communities and the ghosts of misinformation that haunted the corridors of the internet.

The human psyche, a complex mosaic of emotions, responded to Omicron with a kaleidoscope of reactions. Anxiety, a constant companion in the pandemic era, reared its head once more. The fear of the unknown, amplified by the rapid spread of information, became a silent undercurrent that flowed through the consciousness of individuals and communities alike.

Amid the concern, however, resilience emerged as a counterpoint to fear. Communities, battle-hardened by the trials of the past, rallied together in shared determination. Acts of kindness, borne of a collective understanding of vulnerability, became the stitches that wove the fabric of societal response. From mutual aid groups to online support networks, the human spirit, perennial in its ability to adapt, found ways to connect even as physical distances grew.

Public perceptions, a dynamic interplay of information and emotion, set the stage for the unfolding drama of the Omicron era. As individuals grappled with the implications of the new variant, their responses became threads in a tapestry that reflected not only the anxieties of the present but the resilience that would shape the uncertain future.

Epidemiological Insights

Understanding the Characteristics of the Omicron Variant

In the halls of laboratories and the chambers of scientific inquiry, the quest to unravel the mysteries of the Omicron variant took center stage. As the world grappled with the implications of its arrival, scientists embarked on a journey into the microscopic realm, seeking to decipher the genetic code that defined this new player in the ongoing saga of the COVID-19 pandemic.

The genetic sequence of Omicron, a complex arrangement of A, T, C, and G, became the Rosetta Stone for researchers. Every nucleotide, every mutation, held clues to the behavior of the variant, and scientists huddled over their microscopes and computer screens in a collective effort to unveil its secrets.

Initial reports hinted at a constellation of mutations, a genetic fingerprint that distinguished Omicron from its viral predecessors. The spike protein, the very key that the virus used to unlock the cellular door, bore the marks of significant alterations. It was as if nature, in its perpetual dance of adaptation, had choreographed a remix of the viral code.

The significance of these mutations echoed through the scientific community. Questions reverberated in research institutions worldwide: Would Omicron prove more transmissible than its predecessors? Could it evade the immune defenses built by previous infections or vaccinations? What impact might it have on the severity of illness?

The early answers, shrouded in the cautious language of scientific inquiry, hinted at a variant that possessed a unique set of characteristics. Omicron appeared to be highly mutable, a trait that raised concerns about its potential to evade immunity. The virus, it seemed, was playing a game of genetic roulette, spinning its genomic wheel and generating an array of possibilities.

The spike protein mutations, a key focus of attention, suggested a potential increase in transmissibility. It was as if Omicron had acquired a set of keys that allowed it to unlock doors more efficiently, facilitating its entry into human cells. The implications of this heightened transmissibility sent ripples through the public health community, prompting a reevaluation of strategies to curb the spread.

As scientists pieced together the puzzle of Omicron's genetic makeup, a nuanced picture emerged. It was not merely a single mutation but a constellation of changes that collectively altered the virus's characteristics. The scientific lexicon expanded to include terms like "immune escape" and "antigenic drift," each phrase carrying weighty implications for the trajectory of the pandemic.

The virus, ever the elusive adversary, seemed to be engaged in a dance with human immunity. The antibodies forged in the crucible of previous infections and vaccinations faced a formidable opponent in Omicron. The variant's ability to partially evade immunity raised questions about the efficacy of existing vaccines and the potential need for updated formulations.

As the scientific discourse unfolded, it became clear that Omicron was not just a variant; it was a dynamic force that demanded constant vigilance and adaptation. The very essence of its existence lay in the ability to change, to elude the grasp of the immune system and propagate in new environments.

The virus, in its microscopic realm, was scripting a narrative of evolution that mirrored the adaptability of the human societies it traversed.

Expert Opinions and Scientific Perspectives

The unveiling of Omicron's genomic secrets triggered a chorus of expert opinions, a symphony of voices that echoed through media channels, research publications, and public forums. Scientists, armed with data and insights, stepped into the spotlight, becoming the guides navigating society through the uncharted waters of the Omicron era.

In the vast landscape of scientific opinions, there was a nuanced spectrum of perspectives. Some experts, seasoned by years of virological study, approached Omicron with a measured confidence. They emphasized the dynamic nature of viruses, highlighting that mutations were a natural part of the evolutionary dance between pathogens and their hosts.

These voices, grounded in the principles of immunology and virology, urged a perspective tempered by an understanding of the broader context. They reminded the public that the mere presence of mutations did not necessarily translate into increased severity or an insurmountable challenge for existing immunity. It was a call for resilience, a recognition that the scientific community had weathered previous storms and emerged with a deeper understanding of viral dynamics.

Contrastingly, other experts, cognizant of the potential risks posed by Omicron, advocated for a stance of heightened caution. They pointed to the unique combination of mutations, particularly in the spike protein, as a cause for concern. The specter of increased transmissibility and the potential for immune escape raised flags in the minds of health authorities and policymakers.

The divergence in expert opinions, far from sowing confusion, reflected the inherent complexity of the situation. Science, a process of continual inquiry and refinement, thrived on diversity of thought. The debates within the scientific community were not signs of weakness but testaments to the rigor of the inquiry process.

In the public arena, however, the cacophony of expert voices became a double-edged sword. On one hand, it provided a wealth of perspectives for individuals to consider. On the other, it fostered an environment where uncertainty became a breeding ground for anxiety and confusion.

The challenge for the public, amidst this symphony of expert opinions, was to navigate the sea of information with a discerning eye. It required an understanding that scientific inquiry is an iterative process, where hypotheses evolve and consensus emerges over time. The nuances of uncertainty, inherent in any scientific endeavor, demanded a recalibration of expectations and an acknowledgment that answers might be elusive in the immediacy of the moment.

As expert opinions echoed through public discourse, another layer of complexity emerged—the delicate dance between science and policy. Health authorities, entrusted with the responsibility of safeguarding public health, faced the challenge of translating scientific insights into actionable strategies. The evolving nature of the pandemic demanded flexibility in policy-making, a quality often at odds with the desire for definitive answers.

The public, caught in the crossfire of expert opinions and policy decisions, grappled with a dual challenge. On one front, there was the need to digest complex scientific information, often conveyed in technical language. On the other, there was the imperative to navigate the practical implications of this information in daily life—decisions about vaccination, mask-wearing, and social interactions.

Governmental Response

Analyzing How Governments Worldwide Are Addressing the New Variant

The emergence of the Omicron variant was not just a scientific conundrum; it was a call to action for governments worldwide. As news of the new variant rippled across borders, leaders found themselves at the helm of a ship navigating uncharted waters, making decisions that would shape the trajectory of the ongoing pandemic.

The initial response, a delicate ballet of caution and decisiveness, varied from nation to nation. Governments, informed by the lessons of earlier waves, grappled with the challenge of balancing public health imperatives with the socioeconomic realities of their populations. The very nature of the Omicron variant, shrouded in uncertainties, demanded a nimble approach, where policies evolved in tandem with emerging scientific insights.

One of the first arrows in the quiver of governmental response was the reimposition of travel restrictions. The lessons learned from the initial waves of the pandemic had ingrained in policymakers the importance of early action. Airports, once symbols of connectivity, became gatekeepers standing sentinel against the potential influx of Omicron. Travel bans, a tool with both practical and symbolic significance, unfolded as nations sought to shield themselves from the variant's potential reach.

The decision to close borders, however, was not without its complexities. It carried economic implications, disrupting not only international travel but also the global flow of goods and services. Supply chains, already strained by earlier disruptions, faced the specter of new challenges. Governments, in their pursuit of safeguarding public health, were forced to grapple with the delicate dance of protecting lives while mitigating the impact on livelihoods.

Simultaneously, the policy toolkit expanded to include measures such as increased testing and vaccination requirements. The vision of a world where testing was ubiquitous and vaccinations were a shield against severe illness became a cornerstone of governmental strategies. Testing centers, once sporadic and overwhelmed during peaks, multiplied in number, transforming public spaces into arenas of vigilance.

The vaccination narrative, which had been a beacon of hope in earlier chapters of the pandemic, faced a new challenge. The question of vaccine effectiveness against Omicron became a central point of concern. Governments, already engaged in massive vaccination campaigns, found themselves recalibrating strategies based on emerging data. Booster shots, once a topic of discussion, became a focal point in the race to enhance immunity.

Public communication, a linchpin in the machinery of governmental response, became a delicate art. Leaders stepped before cameras and podiums, attempting to convey a sense of reassurance without downplaying the gravity of the situation. The tone of addresses shifted, mirroring the evolving nature of the pandemic. Where once there were messages of triumph over the virus, now there were acknowledgments of the challenges posed by an adversary that seemed to defy prediction.

The intricacies of governmental response were further accentuated by the delicate dance between central authority and regional autonomy. Federal and state governments, provinces and territories—each level of governance faced the challenge of aligning their responses with the unique needs of their populations. Decentralization, once a source of adaptability, became a double-edged sword, with the potential for a patchwork of policies that mirrored the mosaic of a nation.

In this complex landscape, the role of public health agencies and experts became paramount. The faces of epidemiologists and virologists, once confined to scientific journals, became familiar presences in living rooms and virtual spaces. Their voices, laden with the weight of expertise, guided governments in navigating the stormy seas of uncertainty.

The dynamics of governmental response were not confined to the national stage. International collaborations, an undercurrent in the global response to the pandemic, gained renewed significance. Nations, facing a common adversary, engaged in a dance of diplomacy and information-sharing. The World Health Organization, already a linchpin in the fight against the pandemic, found its role further elevated as it coordinated efforts to understand and address the Omicron variant on a global scale.

However, the collaborative spirit was not without its challenges. Vaccine distribution, an issue that had fueled discussions throughout the pandemic, resurfaced with renewed urgency. The global imbalance in vaccine access became a glaring concern as nations with robust vaccination campaigns faced the moral imperative of extending a lifeline to those still grappling with the basics of vaccine coverage.

Economic considerations, always intertwined with public health decisions, took center stage once more. Lockdowns, once a blunt instrument in the arsenal against the virus, faced scrutiny. The delicate balance between protecting lives and preserving livelihoods became a tightrope walk for governments navigating the uncharted terrain of the Omicron era.

As governments worldwide grappled with these multifaceted challenges, a human drama unfolded in the lives of individuals and communities. Policies were not abstract concepts but directives that shaped the contours of daily existence. The closures of borders meant separated families and disrupted plans. Testing requirements translated into lines outside clinics and the uneasy anticipation of results. Vaccine campaigns, once a beacon of hope, became a testament to collective resilience.

Policy Changes and Public Health Measures

Amidst the ebb and flow of governmental response, policy changes and public health measures emerged as the brushstrokes on the canvas of the Omicron era. Lockdowns, once wielded as a last resort, faced a metamorphosis into targeted interventions. The surgical precision required by governments became an art form, attempting to isolate and contain outbreaks without resorting to the sweeping closures of the past.

Public spaces, once the arenas of social interaction, became landscapes transformed by the imperative of physical distancing. Masks, the humble tools of the pandemic era, retained their place in the ensemble of preventive measures. Where the mask had once been a symbol of collective responsibility, it now became a talisman against an adversary that seemed to be testing the limits of our defenses.

Education systems, perennially caught in the crossfire of the pandemic's disruptions, faced renewed challenges. The question of whether to keep schools open or resort to virtual learning became a topic of heated debate. The very essence of education, the connection between students and teachers, faced the threat of unraveling in the face of a microscopic adversary.

The workplace, already transformed by the remote work revolution, faced further adaptations. Hybrid models, once experiments, became the norm as organizations sought to balance productivity with the well-being of their employees. The cubicles and corner offices of yesteryear became relics, replaced by the virtual interconnectedness of a workforce navigating the challenges of the new normal.

Cultural and sporting events, once symbols of communal joy, faced the specter of cancellations and restrictions. The cheers of crowds in stadiums were replaced by the echoes of empty seats. The vibrant tapestry of festivals and gatherings, woven by generations, faced the threat of unraveling as societies grappled with the need for caution.

The intricacies of these policy changes extended beyond the macroscopic lens of governance to the microcosms of individual lives. The closure of a favorite neighborhood cafe, the cancellation of long-awaited travel plans, the postponement of life milestones—each policy decision carried with it the weight of personal stories and shared experiences.

Governments, in their quest to address the Omicron variant, became architects of societal norms. The very fabric of daily life was rewoven by the hands of policymakers, who grappled with the delicate balance between preserving the semblance of normalcy and safeguarding public health.

As the policies unfolded, public compliance became a critical variable in the equation of success. The very measures designed to protect communities were contingent on the

willingness of individuals to adhere to guidelines. Mask mandates, vaccination campaigns, and testing requirements became not just directives from above but a collective pact, a societal contract to navigate the uncertainties of the Omicron era.

Healthcare Systems Under Pressure

Impact on Hospitals and Healthcare Infrastructure

In the unfolding drama of the Omicron era, healthcare systems emerged as the frontline warriors, facing the relentless onslaught of a microscopic adversary. Hospitals, once the sanctuaries of healing, transformed into battlegrounds where the resilience of healthcare professionals clashed with the unpredictability of a virus that seemed to defy conventional wisdom.

The impact on hospitals was multi-faceted, stretching the very fabric of healthcare infrastructure to its limits. Emergency rooms, the first point of contact for the unwell, faced a surge in patient numbers that strained the capacity of even the most robust systems. The cadence of sirens, once a sporadic rhythm in the background, became a constant refrain echoing through the halls of medical facilities.

The challenges were not merely quantitative; they were qualitative, testing the very foundations of healthcare delivery. Intensive care units, the last line of defense against severe illness, faced a critical juncture. Ventilators, once the symbol of life support, became precious commodities in a world where the demand for critical care outstripped the available resources.

The bedrock of healthcare, the dedicated professionals who stood between the virus and its potential victims, faced the weight of emotional and physical exhaustion. Doctors, nurses, and support staff, already scarred by the traumas of earlier waves, found themselves confronting a new chapter that demanded not just clinical expertise but unyielding resilience.

The strain on healthcare personnel was not confined to the walls of hospitals. Ambulance crews, the lifelines connecting communities with care, faced the unenviable task of navigating a landscape where every call carried the potential for exposure. The very act of transporting patients, once routine, became a high-stakes endeavor as paramedics grappled with the challenges of providing care in an environment where the virus seemed to be omnipresent.

The toll on mental health became a silent undercurrent in the narrative of healthcare professionals. Burnout, a phenomenon that had already been a concern in the pre-pandemic era, reached new heights. The constant barrage of cases, the emotional weight of witnessing suffering, and the perpetual uncertainty of the situation became heavy burdens on the shoulders of those tasked with preserving life.

Beyond the immediate frontline, the ripple effects of the strain on healthcare systems extended to elective procedures and routine medical care. Surgeries, once scheduled with precision, faced cancellations as hospitals redirected resources to cope with the demands of the Omicron surge. Routine screenings, the foundation of preventive care, became casualties of a system stretched thin.

The strains on healthcare infrastructure were not confined to the developed world. In resource-limited settings, where healthcare systems were already contending with challenges, the impact of the Omicron variant was amplified. The delicate balance between infectious disease management and the provision of basic healthcare became a tightrope walk, with the potential for cascading effects on maternal and child health, infectious disease control, and overall community well-being.

Strategies to Manage the Surge in Cases

In the face of this multifaceted challenge, healthcare systems worldwide adopted a spectrum of strategies to manage the surge in Omicron cases. The toolkit included both retrospective lessons from earlier waves and novel adaptations forged in the crucible of the evolving pandemic.

One key pillar of the strategy was the expansion of testing capacity. Testing, once a diagnostic tool, became a linchpin in the efforts to trace and contain the spread of the virus. Testing centers, initially concentrated in urban hubs, multiplied to become ubiquitous fixtures in communities. The drive for accessibility became a mantra, with policymakers striving to ensure that testing was not just available but easily reachable for all segments of the population.

Contact tracing, a foundational element in infectious disease control, faced new challenges in the context of Omicron. The variant's heightened transmissibility, coupled with the potential for a shorter incubation period, demanded a recalibration of traditional contact tracing methodologies. Digital solutions, once experimental, gained renewed significance as governments sought to leverage technology for swift and efficient contact identification.

Quarantine and isolation protocols, cornerstones in the containment of infectious diseases, faced adaptations in response to the evolving nature of the pandemic. The concept of quarantine hotels, initially introduced in earlier waves, gained renewed attention as governments sought to manage the influx of cases and minimize the risk of community transmission.

Vaccination campaigns, perennial in the fight against the virus, faced a renewed sense of urgency. Booster shots, once an augmentation to primary vaccination, became a focal point in the race to enhance immunity. Mass vaccination centers, which had become symbols of hope in earlier chapters of the pandemic, saw a resurgence as governments endeavored to boost coverage in the face of the Omicron challenge.

Therapeutic interventions, a critical dimension in the spectrum of care, faced adaptations to address the specific characteristics of the Omicron variant. Antiviral medications, once a topic of research and development, gained prominence as tools to mitigate the severity of illness and reduce the burden on healthcare systems. Monoclonal antibodies, with their potential to neutralize the virus, became valuable assets in the armory against severe disease.

Hospital surge plans, honed through the experiences of previous waves, were activated as healthcare facilities braced for the impact of Omicron. The conversion of non-traditional spaces into temporary medical facilities became a familiar sight, echoing the wartime practices of setting up field hospitals to cope with the influx of casualties.

The role of technology in healthcare underwent a paradigm shift. Telemedicine, once a peripheral option, became a mainstream channel for healthcare delivery. Virtual consultations, already gaining traction, became not just a convenience but a necessity in an era where minimizing physical interactions was a key strategy.

Beyond the immediate response, governments and healthcare authorities engaged in a delicate dance of resource allocation. The procurement of medical supplies, from personal protective equipment to critical care medications, became a logistical challenge. The global demand for such resources, amplified by the simultaneous surges in multiple regions, tested the resilience of supply chains and the diplomatic intricacies of international cooperation.

In the realm of public communication, transparency became both a shield and a vulnerability. Governments, tasked with conveying the gravity of the situation while maintaining public trust, faced the challenge of balancing realism with reassurance. The nuances of scientific uncertainty, inherent in the ever-evolving understanding of the Omicron variant, demanded a delicate touch in public messaging.

As healthcare systems navigated the surge in cases, the importance of public compliance became a recurring theme. The success of strategies hinged on the willingness of individuals to adhere to guidelines, from testing and vaccination to quarantine measures. The narrative of collective responsibility, a cornerstone in the fight against the virus, gained renewed significance.

The challenges faced by healthcare systems were not confined to the present moment; they extended into the realm of future preparedness. Lessons gleaned from the Omicron era would shape the blueprints for pandemic planning and response in the years to come. The imperatives of building resilient healthcare infrastructure, investing in research and development, and fostering international collaborations became keystones in the architecture of future pandemic preparedness.

Impact on Healthcare Professionals and Mental Health Challenges

In the heart of the battle against the Omicron variant were the healthcare professionals—doctors, nurses, paramedics, and support staff—who stood as the human bulwarks against the virus. Their experiences painted a poignant narrative of sacrifice, resilience, and the toll that the pandemic exacted on the human spirit.

The emotional weight of witnessing suffering, the perpetual uncertainty of the situation, and the relentless pace of the pandemic exact

ed a toll on the mental health of healthcare professionals. Burnout, already a concern in the high-stakes world of healthcare, reached new heights. The constant exposure to illness and death became not just a professional challenge but a personal burden that many carried in silence.

The concept of moral injury, a term that gained prominence in the context of healthcare during the pandemic, found resonance in the experiences of those on the frontline. Healthcare professionals, driven by a calling to heal, found themselves confronting situations where the limits of care were defined not by medical capabilities but by resource constraints and the unpredictable nature of the virus.

The erosion of work-life balance, already a concern in the demanding field of healthcare, became a glaring issue. The boundary between professional duty and personal well-being blurred as healthcare professionals grappled with the perpetual demands of the pandemic. Long hours, emotional fatigue, and the constant vigilance required to navigate a high-risk environment became constants in their lives.

Support systems, both within and outside the healthcare setting, played a critical role in the well-being of healthcare professionals. Peer support networks, where individuals could share their experiences and seek solace in the company of those who understood the unique challenges they faced, gained renewed significance. Mental health resources, once relegated to the background, became essential pillars in the framework of support for healthcare professionals.

The impact on mental health extended beyond the immediate frontline to the broader healthcare workforce. Administrative staff, laboratory technicians, and individuals in ancillary roles found themselves navigating the complexities of a high-stress environment. The notion of collective resilience, a thread that wove through the experiences of healthcare professionals, became a rallying point for teams facing the challenges of the Omicron era.

The psychological toll on healthcare professionals reverberated beyond the confines of the hospital. Families, witnessing the strains on their loved ones, became silent witnesses to the emotional burdens carried by those who dedicated themselves to the care of others. Spouses, children, and parents found themselves navigating a delicate dance of support, attempting to provide solace in a time of collective turmoil.

The mental health challenges faced by healthcare professionals also highlighted the imperative of systemic changes. The stigma surrounding mental health in the medical profession, often a barrier to seeking help, faced scrutiny. Conversations about mental health, once confined to private spaces, gained visibility as the importance of addressing the emotional well-being of healthcare professionals became a central theme in the discourse surrounding pandemic response.

Beyond the immediate challenges, the experiences of healthcare professionals during the Omicron era sparked reflections on the broader societal dynamics that shaped the landscape of healthcare. The acknowledgment of the human toll on those in the medical profession became a catalyst for conversations about systemic issues, from workforce shortages to the need for comprehensive mental health support.

As we navigate the chapters that follow, the human narrative of healthcare professionals will remain at the forefront. Their stories, etched with the indelible marks of sacrifice and resilience, serve as a poignant reminder of the complexities faced by those on the frontline of the Omicron era.

Impact on Vulnerable Populations and Health Inequities

In the intricate tapestry of the Omicron era, the impact on vulnerable populations became a chapter that underscored the existing fault lines of health inequities. Communities already facing barriers to healthcare access, socioeconomic disparities, and systemic challenges found themselves disproportionately affected by the new variant.

The concept of vulnerability extended beyond the traditional metrics of age or pre-existing health conditions. Socioeconomic factors, including income disparities and access to resources, played a pivotal role in shaping the differential impact of the Omicron variant. The virus, seemingly indiscriminate in its transmission, found fertile ground in the vulnerabilities that were already embedded in the fabric of society.

Marginalized communities, often at the intersection of multiple layers of vulnerability, faced compounded challenges. Access to healthcare, a perennial concern, became a critical factor in the ability to navigate the complexities of the Omicron era. The very systems designed to protect public health, in their strained state, inadvertently exacerbated existing health inequities.

The role of social determinants of health, long acknowledged as influential factors in health outcomes, gained renewed prominence. Housing conditions, employment precarity, and the lack of access to education became not just markers of social disadvantage but determinants of susceptibility to the virus. Vulnerable populations, already navigating a landscape of systemic challenges, found themselves grappling with the additional burden of a microscopic adversary.

The digital divide, often framed in the context of access to technology, gained new dimensions in the era of Omicron. Telemedicine, once heralded as a solution for healthcare accessibility, faced the stark reality that not all communities had equal access to the internet or the devices required for virtual consultations. The disparities in access to healthcare, already a concern, became glaring issues that demanded attention.

The economic impact on vulnerable populations, already under the shadow of pre-existing disparities, faced a perfect storm in the Omicron era. Lockdowns, restrictions, and disruptions to daily life bore a heavier burden on communities with limited financial resources. The choice between following public health guidelines and meeting basic needs became a precarious balance for many individuals and families.

The impact on mental health in vulnerable populations became a parallel narrative that unfolded against the backdrop of healthcare challenges. The stressors of economic uncertainty, concerns about housing stability, and the perpetual anxiety of navigating a high-risk environment compounded the mental health challenges faced by vulnerable communities. The existing mental health disparities, often linked to socioeconomic factors, gained new dimensions in the era of Omicron.

Access to healthcare services, a cornerstone in the fight against the virus, faced challenges in the context of vulnerable populations. The strains on healthcare infrastructure, coupled with pre-existing barriers to access, created a perfect storm that hindered the ability of communities already facing health inequities to seek timely and adequate care.

Vaccine access, a linchpin in the global strategy against the virus, faced hurdles in reaching vulnerable populations. The disparities in vaccine coverage, influenced by factors such as geography, income, and education, became emblematic of the broader challenges in achieving health equity. The imperative of addressing vaccine hesitancy, often rooted in historical mistrust and systemic injustices, gained renewed significance.

Community engagement and public health outreach became critical elements in addressing health inequities during the Omicron era. The very communities that faced heightened vulnerabilities were often the ones where trust in public health messaging needed rebuilding. Grassroots initiatives, culturally competent outreach, and partnerships with community leaders became essential strategies in bridging the gaps in health communication.

The experiences of vulnerable populations during the Omicron era were not just stories of hardship; they were narratives of resilience. Community-led initiatives, mutual aid networks, and the strength forged in the crucible of shared challenges became testaments to the human spirit. Vulnerable communities, often defined by their ability to adapt and support one another, navigated the complexities of the Omicron era with a sense of collective determination.

Impact on Children and Education Systems

As the Omicron variant unfolded its chapters, the impact on children and education systems became a poignant narrative that echoed through the hallways of schools and the homes of families. The pandemic, already a disruptive force, faced a new chapter that tested the resilience of the youngest members of society and the systems designed to nurture their growth.

The closure of schools, a measure adopted to curb the spread of the virus, became a defining feature of the Omicron era. Classrooms, once vibrant spaces of learning and social interaction, transformed into echoes of silence. The laughter of children, the hum of discussions, and the cadence of teachers became memories as education systems grappled with the challenges of providing continuity in the midst of uncertainty.

Remote learning, a phenomenon that had gained prominence in the earlier waves of the pandemic, faced new adaptations. The very notion of education shifted from the physical confines of classrooms to the virtual realm. The screens of laptops and tablets became windows into the world of learning, connecting students and teachers in a digital landscape that bridged physical distances but introduced new challenges.

The digital divide, a pre-existing concern in education, became a stark reality in the era of Omicron. Not all students had equal access to devices, high-speed internet, or conducive home environments for learning. The disparities in access to technology, often linked to socioeconomic factors, became fault lines that shaped the ability of students to engage with remote education.

The role of parents in the educational landscape underwent a transformation. Homes, once sanctuaries of family life, became makeshift classrooms where parents juggled the roles of caregivers, educators, and often remote workers. The challenges of balancing professional responsibilities with the demands of supporting children in their educational journey became a daily reality for many families.

The psychological impact on children, often resilient but not immune to the stresses of the pandemic, gained attention. The absence of the traditional school environment, with its routines, peer interactions, and extracurricular activities, became a void in the lives of young learners. The isolation from friends and the disruptions to familiar routines carried implications for social and emotional development.

Children with special educational needs, already navigating a landscape of unique challenges, faced compounded difficulties in the context of remote learning. The personalized support provided in educational settings became challenging to replicate in the virtual realm. The question of how to address the diverse needs of students with varying learning styles and abilities became a central theme in the discourse surrounding education during the Omicron era.

The impact on educational milestones, from graduations to transitions between school levels, became a shared experience for students around the world. The symbolism of these rites of passage, once marked by ceremonies and celebrations, faced adaptations in the context of social distancing and restrictions on gatherings.

As schools navigated the challenges of the Omicron era, educators emerged as unsung heroes in the narrative of resilience. The pivot to remote learning demanded not just technical adaptability but a fundamental shift in teaching methodologies. Teachers, often navigating their own challenges in the context of the pandemic, became architects of innovative solutions to engage students in the virtual realm.

The reimagining of assessments and examinations became a critical element in education systems worldwide. The traditional models of standardized testing, already facing scrutiny in the pre-pandemic era, encountered new complexities in the context of remote and hybrid learning. The question of how to fairly and accurately assess student progress became a topic of widespread discussion and experimentation.

The reopening of schools, a beacon of hope in the narrative of the Omicron era, faced complexities in the context of ongoing uncertainties. The delicate balance between providing a safe environment for students and staff and the imperative of resuming in-person learning became a central theme in the discourse surrounding education.

Beyond the immediate challenges, the experiences of children during the Omicron era sparked reflections on the broader societal dynamics that shaped the landscape of education. The question of how to build resilient education systems that can withstand the shocks of future disruptions became a central theme in discussions about the post-pandemic era.

Navigating Everyday Life

The Fabric of Daily Existence in the Omicron Era

In the intricate dance between the virus and society, the chapters of everyday life unfolded against the backdrop of the Omicron variant. The nuances of human interactions, the rhythms of work and leisure, and the very fabric of daily existence faced adaptations in the face of an evolving reality that seemed to rewrite the rules of normalcy.

Shifts in Work Dynamics

The workplace, once a physical hub where colleagues gathered and ideas flowed in the shared spaces of offices, underwent a metamorphosis. The remote work revolution, sparked by earlier waves of the pandemic, gained permanence as organizations embraced hybrid models. The cubicles and corner offices of yesteryear became relics, replaced by the virtual interconnectedness of a workforce navigating the challenges of the new normal.

For many, the home, once a sanctuary separate from the demands of professional life, became an extension of the workplace. Dining tables became desks, living rooms transformed into meeting spaces, and the rhythms of family life intertwined with the cadence of virtual meetings. The boundaries between professional duties and personal spaces blurred as individuals sought to balance the demands of work with the realities of daily life.

The implications of this shift in work dynamics were far-reaching. Commutes, once a staple of daily routines, became artifacts of a bygone era. The hustle and bustle of rush hour, the shared journeys on public transportation, and the solo drives in the solitude of personal vehicles underwent a hiatus. The very notion of commuting, once synonymous with the beginning and end of the workday, faced adaptations in a world where the concept of a physical office became more fluid.

The impact of remote work extended beyond the logistical shifts to the social dynamics of the workplace. Watercooler conversations, once the informal spaces where camaraderie and idea exchange flourished, faced a virtual transformation. The rituals of birthday celebrations, team-building activities, and the spontaneous interactions that fueled workplace culture underwent adaptations in the context of screens and pixels.

For some, the transition to remote work brought newfound flexibility. The ability to design workdays around personal rhythms, to be present for family moments, and to escape the rigidity of traditional office hours became elements of a new work-life balance. The autonomy afforded by remote work became a source of empowerment for individuals who found themselves liberated from the constraints of physical office spaces.

However, the utopia of remote work was not universal. Many faced the challenges of isolation, the blurring of boundaries between work and personal life, and the absence of the social fabric that had woven through the daily routines of office life. The camaraderie built through shared challenges, the mentorship that flourished in face-to-face interactions, and the intangible elements of workplace culture faced erosion in the context of virtual spaces.

The concept of a digital nomad, once a niche lifestyle choice, gained mainstream attention as individuals sought the flexibility to work from locations beyond the confines of their home cities. The rise of co-living and co-working spaces in picturesque locales became symbols of a lifestyle that blended professional responsibilities with the pursuit of adventure and a sense of community.

As organizations grappled with the challenges and opportunities presented by the new dynamics of work, the very essence of leadership faced adaptations. The traditional models of supervising and managing teams, built on physical presence and observable cues, encountered new challenges in the context of virtual collaborations. The question of how to foster a sense of cohesion, provide mentorship, and nurture professional growth in a digital landscape became a central theme in the discourse on leadership.

Transformations in Social Interactions

The contours of social interactions, once defined by the warmth of handshakes, hugs, and shared spaces, faced a redefinition. The handshake, a universal gesture of greeting and agreement, became a relic of the past as societies grappled with the imperative of physical distancing. The very act of greeting, once an instinctive part of human interactions, faced adaptations in a world where proximity carried the weight of potential risk.

The dynamics of gatherings and celebrations underwent transformations. Birthday parties, weddings, and festive gatherings, once marked by the conviviality of shared spaces, faced the specter of restrictions and the imperative of caution. The very essence of communal joy, the cheers of crowds in stadiums, the vibrant tapestry of festivals, and the simple pleasure of shared meals underwent adaptations in a world where the virus seemed to be an uninvited guest in every gathering.

The etiquette of social interactions gained new dimensions. The mask, once a symbol of collective responsibility, became a constant companion in public spaces. The very act of wearing a mask became not just a preventive measure but a statement of solidarity—a tangible expression of the shared commitment to safeguarding community health.

Restaurants and cafes, once the bustling hubs of social life, faced adaptations. The traditional experience of dining out, with its conviviality, shared plates, and the ambient hum of conversations, underwent changes. Tables spaced apart, capacity restrictions, and the imperative of contactless transactions became elements of the new dining experience.

The very essence of travel, once synonymous with exploration and adventure, faced adaptations. Airports, once symbols of connectivity, became gatekeepers standing sentinel against the potential influx of the virus. The thrill of boarding a plane, the shared excitement of discovering new destinations, and the serendipity of chance encounters faced the realities of travel restrictions, testing requirements, and the uncertainty of evolving situations.

The impact on cultural and sporting events became a poignant chapter in the narrative of social life. The cheers of crowds in stadiums were replaced by the echoes of empty seats. The vibrant tapestry of festivals and gatherings, woven by generations, faced the threat of unraveling as societies grappled with the need for caution.

The digital realm, once a supplementary space for social interactions, gained renewed significance. Virtual gatherings, whether through video calls or social media platforms, became lifelines connecting individuals across physical distances. The celebration of milestones, the sharing of everyday moments, and the collective experience of virtual events became central elements in the repertoire of social interactions.

Dating and romantic relationships faced adaptations in the context of the pandemic. The nuances of courtship, the shared experiences of exploring new places, and the simple joy of physical closeness faced challenges in a world where the very act of proximity carried considerations of risk. Dating apps, once a channel for meeting new people, became not just tools for connecting but platforms for navigating conversations about health and safety.

The impact on social interactions extended beyond the external dimensions of gatherings and gestures. The emotional nuances of relationships, the unspoken language of facial expressions, and the subtleties of non-verbal cues faced adaptations in a world where masks concealed smiles and virtual interactions often flattened the richness of in-person connections.

Navigating Public Spaces and Services

The very concept of public spaces underwent adaptations in the Omicron era. Parks, once havens of outdoor recreation and community gatherings, became landscapes where physical distancing was the order of the day. The simple pleasure of a leisurely stroll or a picnic faced considerations of spacing and the imperative of avoiding crowded areas.

Public transportation, once the arteries that connected communities, faced transformations. The ebb and flow of commuters, the shared spaces of buses and trains, and the very essence of the daily commute underwent changes. The considerations of safety, the spacing of seats, and the imperatives of hygiene became central themes in the experience of public transportation.

The retail landscape, once marked by the tactile experience of browsing shelves and the shared spaces of malls, faced adaptations. The

surge in online shopping, driven by convenience and the imperative of contactless transactions, became a defining feature of consumer behavior. The very act of entering stores, once a routine part of daily life, became a strategic decision weighed against considerations of safety.

The very essence of healthcare interactions faced transformations. The waiting rooms, once spaces where individuals sought care for a myriad of health concerns, became landscapes where caution and distancing were paramount. Telemedicine, once a supplementary channel for healthcare delivery, gained permanence as a mainstream option for consultations.

The education landscape faced adaptations in the realm of public spaces. Classrooms, once vibrant spaces of learning and interaction, underwent changes to accommodate the imperatives of physical distancing. The very act of entering educational institutions, once marked by the energy of students converging in shared spaces, faced considerations of safety and adherence to protocols.

The very notion of public events, from cultural performances to community gatherings, faced challenges. The organizers of events, once focused on the logistics of creating memorable experiences, now grappled with the complexities of ensuring safety, implementing protocols, and navigating the uncertainties of evolving situations.

The impact on essential services became a critical dimension in the narrative of navigating public spaces. Grocery stores, once bustling hubs of daily life, faced challenges in maintaining supply chains, implementing safety measures, and adapting to shifts in consumer behavior. The very act of purchasing essentials, once marked by the routine of browsing aisles, faced considerations of efficiency and safety.

Mental Health and Coping Mechanisms

In the ebb and flow of everyday life, the mental health of individuals became a central theme. The strains of uncertainty, the perpetual vigilance required to navigate a high-risk environment, and the adaptations to changing norms carried implications for the well-being of individuals.

The isolation faced by many, whether due to remote work, physical distancing measures, or the absence of social gatherings, became a silent undercurrent in the human narrative. Loneliness, often a silent companion, gained visibility as individuals navigated the challenges of extended periods without the familiar rhythms of social interactions.

The impact on mental health extended beyond the dimensions of isolation. Anxiety, fueled by the uncertainties of the pandemic and the perpetual influx of information, became a prevalent theme. The very act of navigating public spaces, once routine, became tinged with considerations of risk and the need for constant vigilance.

Depression, often linked to the challenges of adapting to new norms and the disruptions to daily life, became a tangible concern. The loss of routines, the uncertainties of the future, and the erosion of familiar anchors in the landscape of everyday life became factors that weighed on the mental well-being of individuals.

The coping mechanisms adopted by individuals became varied and personal. Some turned to hobbies, whether rediscovering old passions or exploring new ones, as a means of finding solace in the midst of uncertainty. The pursuit of creative outlets, from artistic endeavors to culinary experiments, became not just leisure activities but therapeutic interventions.

Physical activity, once woven into the routines of daily life through gym sessions, sports, or outdoor activities, faced adaptations. The rise of home workouts, virtual fitness classes, and the embrace of outdoor activities became not just alternatives but essential elements in the pursuit of physical and mental well-being.

Mindfulness and mental health practices gained renewed attention. The pursuit of meditation, the exploration of mindfulness techniques, and the embrace of holistic approaches to well-being became not just trends but integral components of the toolkit for navigating the challenges of the Omicron era.

The role of social connections in mental health became a central theme. Virtual gatherings, whether through video calls or online platforms, became lifelines connecting individuals across distances. The support networks of friends and family, often the pillars of resilience in challenging times, gained renewed significance.

Professional support for mental health, once a stigmatized topic, gained visibility as organizations recognized the importance of employee well-being. Employee assistance programs, mental health resources, and initiatives focused on fostering a culture of well-being in the workplace became integral elements in the discourse on organizational priorities.

The impact on children's mental health became a poignant chapter in the narrative of everyday life. The disruptions to routines, the challenges of adapting to remote learning, and the absence of familiar social interactions carried implications for the emotional well-being of young learners. The role of parents, educators, and support systems in nurturing the mental health of children gained renewed attention.

Resilience and Community Spirit

The Heartbeat of Resilience

In the tapestry of the Omicron era, the threads of resilience woven by individuals and communities became a defining motif. The human spirit, often tested by adversity, revealed its capacity to endure, adapt, and find strength in the face of unprecedented challenges.

Individual Acts of Resilience

At the heart of the narrative were the individual stories of resilience—personal sagas of triumph, perseverance, and the unwavering commitment to navigate the complexities of the Omicron era. These stories unfolded in the daily routines, the moments of solitude, and the myriad decisions made by individuals facing the uncertainties of a world transformed by the virus.

The essential workers, from healthcare professionals to grocery store employees, emerged as unsung heroes in the tapestry of resilience. Their commitment to duty, the sacrifices made to safeguard the well-being of others, and the perseverance shown in the face of adversity became symbols of the indomitable human spirit. The applause from balconies, the gestures of gratitude, and the shared recognition of their contributions became threads in the narrative of communal resilience.

Parents, navigating the complexities of remote work, homeschooling, and the perpetual demands of caregiving, exemplified resilience in everyday life. The juggling act of balancing professional responsibilities with the needs of children, the creativity in finding new ways to create moments of joy, and the unspoken sacrifices made for the well-being of families became chapters in the story of parental resilience.

Individuals facing the strains of isolation found innovative ways to connect and support one another. Virtual book clubs, online support groups, and digital communities became lifelines, fostering a sense of connection in a world where physical distancing was imperative. The human need for social interactions, expressed through screens and pixels, became a testament to the adaptive nature of the human spirit.

Entrepreneurs and small business owners, grappling with the economic impact of the pandemic, displayed resilience in the face of uncertainty. The pivot to online platforms, the creative adaptations to changing consumer behaviors, and the collaborative spirit within business communities became elements of the entrepreneurial narrative. The survival of local businesses, often embedded in the fabric of communities, became a collective triumph.

The pursuit of personal growth and learning became a common theme in the stories of individual resilience. Individuals rediscovered old passions, embarked on new educational pursuits, and explored avenues for self-improvement. The pursuit of knowledge, whether as a form of distraction, a means of empowerment, or a source of solace, became a pathway to resilience.

The role of humor and creativity in navigating adversity became a recurring theme. Memes, satirical content, and online humor became not just sources of entertainment but coping mechanisms in a world where the weight of challenges could feel overwhelming. The ability to find laughter in the midst of difficulties became a reflection of the human capacity to transform moments of hardship into opportunities for resilience.

Community Bonds and Collective Strength

The collective strength of communities emerged as a powerful force in the narrative of resilience. Whether defined by geographical proximity, shared interests, or cultural bonds, communities became pillars of support, connection, and shared resilience.

Neighborhoods transformed into networks of solidarity. Mutual aid groups, formed organically or through organized efforts, became lifelines for individuals facing challenges such as isolation, the inability to access essentials, or the need for emotional support. The simple acts of checking in on neighbors, sharing resources, and offering assistance became integral elements in the communal narrative of resilience.

Volunteerism and community service gained renewed prominence. Individuals, motivated by a sense of responsibility and a desire to contribute to the collective well-being, engaged in a myriad of activities to support those in need. Food drives, mask-making initiatives, and assistance for vulnerable populations became tangible expressions of community resilience.

Cultural and religious communities adapted their traditions to navigate the challenges of the Omicron era. Virtual religious services, online cultural events, and digital celebrations became ways for communities to stay connected and uphold traditions while adhering to safety measures. The resilience of cultural identity and the ability to find meaning in shared rituals became sources of strength.

Educational communities, from schools to universities, exemplified resilience in the face of disruptions. Educators, students, and parents collaborated to navigate the challenges of remote learning, adapting curricula, and finding innovative ways to maintain a sense of continuity in educational pursuits. The shared commitment to the importance of learning and the resilience displayed in the pursuit of knowledge became foundational elements in the educational narrative.

The role of social media in fostering community spirit became evident. Online platforms, often criticized for fostering disconnection, became conduits for the expression of support, the sharing of resources, and the amplification of positive initiatives. Hashtags, trends, and challenges became not just virtual phenomena but tools for mobilizing collective action and fostering a sense of shared resilience.

Community leaders, whether formal or informal, played a pivotal role in guiding their constituencies through the challenges of the Omicron era. The communication of accurate information, the provision of support networks, and the ability to inspire a sense of collective purpose became hallmarks of effective leadership. The resilience of communities often mirrored the strength of their leaders in navigating the complexities of the pandemic.

The concept of "community immunity," extending beyond the realm of vaccination, gained significance. Communities recognized that the well-being of each individual was intertwined with the well-being of the collective. The narrative of collective responsibility, expressed through adherence to public health guidelines, vaccination campaigns, and support for vulnerable populations, became a foundational element in the resilience of communities.

Creative Expressions of Resilience

Art, in its various forms, became a poignant expression of resilience during the Omicron era. Creativity served not only as a form of personal expression but also as a medium for conveying shared experiences, fostering connection, and inspiring hope.

The arts, from visual to performing arts, became channels for navigating and expressing the complexities of the human experience. Artists found inspiration in the challenges of the pandemic, creating works that spoke to the resilience of individuals and communities. Paintings, sculptures, and installations became visual narratives that captured the nuances of the Omicron era.

Literature became a mirror reflecting the human experience during the pandemic. Authors, poets, and storytellers penned works that explored themes of resilience, adaptation, and the indomitable spirit of individuals. The written word became a vessel for preserving

the stories of the Omicron era, offering insights into the human condition in times of crisis.

Music, with its universal language, became a source of solace and inspiration. Musicians composed pieces that reflected the emotional landscape of the pandemic, from the challenges faced to the triumphs celebrated. Virtual concerts, online collaborations, and the sharing of musical creations became not just entertainment but expressions of the collective resilience of societies.

Film and documentary projects delved into the human stories of resilience. Filmmakers captured the narratives of individuals on the frontlines, communities navigating challenges, and the various dimensions of the human experience during the pandemic. Cinematic expressions became not just reflections of reality but catalysts for conversations about the resilience needed in the face of unprecedented challenges.

Photography served as a visual chronicle of the Omicron era. Photographers documented the everyday lives of individuals, the moments of connection in a physically distanced world, and the expressions of resilience in the faces of people. Photojournalism became a powerful tool for conveying the stories of individuals and communities grappling with the realities of the pandemic.

Embracing the Dawn of Hope

In the evolving narrative of the Omicron era, a chapter of hope and renewal began to unfold. As the world navigated the challenges of the variant, the collective resilience of individuals and communities laid the groundwork for a sense of optimism and the prospect of a brighter future.

Vaccination as a Beacon of Hope

The advent of vaccines marked a pivotal moment in the trajectory of the pandemic. Vaccination campaigns, once aspirations, became tangible initiatives that offered a beacon of hope. The collaboration between scientists, pharmaceutical companies, and global health organizations resulted in the development and distribution of vaccines that held the promise of protection against severe illness and the potential for returning to a semblance of normalcy.

The vaccination rollout became a momentous chapter in the Omicron era. Individuals from diverse backgrounds, spanning continents and cultures, rolled up their sleeves to receive doses of protection. Vaccination centers, once symbols of collective vulnerability, transformed into hubs of hope. The air buzzed with a sense of anticipation and the collective recognition that each jab represented a step toward overcoming the challenges posed by the virus.

The concept of herd immunity, once an abstract notion, gained practical significance. Communities recognized that the well-being of each individual was interconnected with the well-being of the collective. The narrative of shared responsibility and the understanding that widespread vaccination was a key to safeguarding community health became central themes in the discourse on pandemic response.

Vaccine hesitancy, a challenge that had to be addressed with empathy and understanding, became a focus of public health campaigns. The narratives shifted from the mechanics of vaccination to the stories of individuals who, once hesitant, found the courage to embrace the vaccine. Personal testimonials, shared through various mediums, became powerful tools for building confidence and dispelling myths surrounding vaccination.

The global efforts to ensure equitable vaccine distribution became a crucial aspect of the narrative of hope. The acknowledgment that the pandemic could only be truly overcome through a collective, worldwide response prompted initiatives to make vaccines accessible to all, regardless of geographical location or economic status. The realization that no one is safe until everyone is safe underscored the interconnectedness of the global community.

The achievement of significant vaccination coverage brought about changes in public health guidelines. Restrictions began to ease as communities achieved milestones in vaccination rates. The return to in-person gatherings, the reopening of businesses and educational institutions, and the gradual resumption of everyday activities became tangible expressions of the progress made in the fight against the virus.

Adaptations in Work and Education

The workplace, having undergone a radical transformation in response to the pandemic, faced a new chapter in the era of hope and renewal. Organizations grappled with decisions about the future of remote work, hybrid models, and the physical spaces that once defined the professional landscape. The lessons learned during the Omicron era prompted reflections on work dynamics, the importance of flexibility, and the value of employee well-being.

The return to physical offices became a symbolic act of resilience and adaptation. Organizations, recognizing the significance of in-person interactions for collaboration, innovation, and team building, navigated the complexities of reestablishing a physical presence. The hybrid work model, blending remote and in-office work, became a strategy that aimed to combine the benefits of flexibility with the advantages of face-to-face collaboration.

Leadership in the post-Omicron workplace faced new dimensions. The challenges of fostering a cohesive team in a hybrid environment, prioritizing employee well-being, and adapting to the evolving expectations of the workforce became central themes. The understanding that the workplace had undergone a fundamental shift prompted leaders to explore innovative approaches to team building, mentorship, and professional development.

The education landscape, having weathered disruptions in the face of the Omicron variant, looked toward a future marked by renewal. Educational institutions embraced lessons learned from remote learning, incorporating technological tools and strategies for flexible educational delivery. The resilience displayed by educators, students, and parents during the challenging times became a source of inspiration for reimagining the future of education.

In-person learning experiences regained prominence as schools and universities adapted to the new normal. The physical classrooms, once vacant, echoed with the sounds of discussions, laughter, and the pursuit of knowledge. The return to on-campus education marked a significant step toward restoring the vibrancy of the educational experience.

The integration of technology in education became a lasting legacy of the Omicron era. Online learning platforms, virtual classrooms, and digital resources became integral components of the educational toolkit. The understanding that technology could enhance accessibility, flexibility, and the overall quality of education prompted a reevaluation of traditional educational models.

The impact of the pandemic on students' mental health and well-being prompted a renewed focus on holistic support systems within educational institutions. The recognition that students needed not only academic but also emotional and social support became a central theme. Initiatives aimed at promoting mental health awareness, providing counseling services, and fostering a sense of community gained renewed importance.

Cultural and Social Reconnections

Cultural and social reconnections became a poignant aspect of the era of hope and renewal. The arts, having served as expressions of resilience, now became mediums for celebrating the return of communal experiences. Cultural events, performances, and exhibitions once postponed or adapted to virtual formats, found their way back to physical venues.

The resumption of live music events became a symbol of the return to normalcy. Concert venues, once silent, echoed with the sounds of music and the cheers of audiences. Musicians, long deprived of the energy of live performances, found inspiration in the shared joy of in-person interactions. Festivals, both large and small, became gatherings that celebrated the resilience of cultural traditions.

The reopening of theaters and cinemas marked a renaissance for the performing arts. Audiences, once confined to virtual screens, returned to the shared experience of live performances. The laughter, tears, and applause once again became integral components of the cultural landscape. The resilience of artists and the enduring nature of cultural expressions became powerful symbols of the human spirit.

Social interactions underwent a renaissance as communities embraced the return to gatherings. The handshake, once replaced by distant waves or nods, regained its place as a universal gesture of greeting. Shared meals, hugs, and the simple joy of being in close proximity to loved ones became cherished experiences. The reconnection with friends, family, and communities marked a chapter of healing and renewal.

The impact on travel, once marked by restrictions and uncertainties, began

to transform. Airports, once silent, bustled with the excitement of travelers embarking on journeys. The shared thrill of exploring new destinations, the joy of reuniting with loved ones separated by distance, and the serendipity of chance encounters once again became hallmarks of the travel experience.

The hospitality industry, having weathered the challenges of lockdowns and restrictions, faced a resurgence. Restaurants, cafes, and hotels, once marked by empty tables and vacant rooms, welcomed back patrons. The shared experiences of dining out, the conviviality of shared spaces, and the exploration of culinary delights became central elements in the narrative of cultural and social renewal.

Environmental Considerations and Sustainable Practices

The Omicron era prompted reflections on the interconnectedness of human health, environmental well-being, and sustainable practices. Communities recognized the importance of adopting practices that not only safeguarded public health but also contributed to the resilience of the planet.

The experiences of reduced human activity during lockdowns prompted reflections on environmental impact. Cleaner air, reduced carbon emissions, and the flourishing of natural habitats during periods of reduced human activity became testaments to the profound impact of human behaviors on the environment. The understanding that a balance could be struck between human activities and environmental health gained traction.

Sustainable practices, once seen as choices made by environmentally conscious individuals, gained mainstream attention. Businesses, communities, and individuals explored ways to reduce their carbon footprint, embrace renewable energy sources, and contribute to the preservation of biodiversity. The collective recognition that individual actions, when multiplied, could have a significant impact on environmental sustainability became a driving force for change.

Urban planning and development faced considerations of creating spaces that prioritized both human well-being and environmental health. The design of cities, buildings, and public spaces began to integrate concepts of sustainability, green infrastructure, and the promotion of healthier lifestyles. The understanding that a harmonious coexistence between human activities and the environment was essential for long-term resilience prompted a shift in planning paradigms.

Resilient Communities for a Sustainable Future

The era of hope and renewal laid the foundation for building resilient communities with an eye toward a sustainable future. The lessons learned from the challenges of the Omicron era prompted communities to explore innovative approaches to collective well-being, environmental stewardship, and the cultivation of a sense of shared responsibility.

Community resilience became synonymous with preparedness for future challenges. The recognition that resilience was not just a response to crises but a continuous effort to build capacity, adaptability, and cohesion prompted communities to invest in initiatives that strengthened social bonds, diversified resources, and fostered a culture of collaboration.

The role of technology in building resilient communities gained prominence.

Digital platforms became tools for communication, coordination, and the dissemination of information during times of crisis. The understanding that technology could bridge gaps, connect individuals, and provide essential services prompted communities to embrace digital solutions as integral components of their resilience strategies.

Local economies, having faced disruptions during the Omicron era, became focal points for building resilience. The support for small businesses, the cultivation of local industries, and the recognition of the importance of self-sufficiency in essential goods and services became central themes. Communities explored ways to enhance economic resilience while prioritizing ethical and sustainable practices.

Community-based healthcare initiatives gained renewed importance. The understanding that health is a collective responsibility prompted communities to invest in healthcare infrastructure, preventive measures, and support systems for vulnerable populations. The pursuit of health equity, where access to healthcare is not determined by socioeconomic factors, became a cornerstone of resilient communities.

Education, as a pillar of community resilience, underwent transformations. The integration of technology, flexible learning models, and a focus on holistic development became priorities. Communities recognized that an educated and adaptable populace was key to navigating the challenges of an ever-evolving world.

The role of community leaders in guiding resilient communities became paramount. Leaders who prioritized inclusivity, transparency, and collaboration found resonance with their constituencies. The understanding that effective leadership was not just about crisis management but also about long-term vision and community well-being shaped the narratives of resilient communities.

As communities reflected on the lessons learned from the Omicron era, the imperative of cultivating a culture of empathy and compassion emerged. Resilient communities recognized the importance of supporting one another through challenges, acknowledging individual differences, and fostering a sense of belonging. The narrative of hope and renewal became intertwined with the commitment to creating communities where every member felt valued and supported.

Looking Toward the Future

As we navigate the chapters that follow, the theme of hope and renewal will continue to evolve. The stories of individuals, communities, and the collective aspirations for a sustainable and resilient future will guide the narrative. In the face of challenges, the human spirit remains indomitable, and the shared journey toward a brighter tomorrow becomes a testament to the capacity for adaptation, collaboration, and the pursuit of a better world.

The Lingering Shadows of Adversity

As the world moved into the post-Omicron era, the challenges faced during the pandemic continued to cast lingering shadows. The intricate tapestry of human experiences revealed not only the triumphs but also the ongoing struggles that persisted in the wake of the variant. From the repercussions on mental health to the reshaping of global dynamics, the narrative unfolded in complex and nuanced ways.

Mental Health in the Aftermath

The echoes of the pandemic reverberated in the realm of mental health. Individuals, having weathered the uncertainties and disruptions of the Omicron era, grappled with the aftermath on emotional well-being. The strains of prolonged stress, the lingering effects of isolation, and the collective trauma experienced globally underscored the need for sustained attention to mental health.

Anxiety, a companion through the uncertainties of the pandemic, persisted for many. The gradual return to pre-pandemic activities brought with it a complex tapestry of emotions—excitement, apprehension, and a heightened awareness of one's surroundings. The challenges of navigating crowded spaces, resuming social interactions, and reconciling with the changes in the world became sources of anxiety for individuals adjusting to the evolving normalcy.

Depression, a shadow that had loomed over the Omicron era, continued to cast its influence. The disruptions to routines, the loss of familiar anchors, and the enduring uncertainties about the future contributed to a sense of melancholy for some. The process of rebuilding lives, careers, and social connections became a journey marked by both resilience and the acknowledgment of the emotional toll exacted by the pandemic.

Grief, a companion to the losses experienced during the Omicron era, took on new dimensions in the aftermath. The collective mourning for lives lost, the missed milestones, and the societal shifts that reshaped the familiar landscape became elements of a grieving process that extended beyond the immediate impact of the variant. The complexities of grieving in a world that was simultaneously healing and adapting posed unique challenges for individuals and communities.

The impact on children's mental health remained a critical consideration. The disruptions to education, the changes in social dynamics, and the uncertainties experienced during the pandemic continued to influence the emotional well-being of young learners. The role of parents, educators, and support systems in nurturing the mental health of children gained renewed attention as societies grappled with the long-term effects on the younger generation.

The stigma surrounding mental health, though gradually diminishing, persisted as a barrier to seeking support. The narratives of resilience, adaptation, and community spirit coexisted with the stories of individuals silently navigating the challenges of mental health. The importance of normalizing conversations about mental well-being, fostering supportive environments, and ensuring access to mental health resources remained central themes in the ongoing narrative.

Economic Transformations and Inequalities

The economic landscape, having faced seismic shifts during the Omicron era, continued to evolve in the post-variant world. The repercussions of lockdowns, disruptions to global supply chains, and changes in consumer behavior left indelible marks on economies at local and global scales. As societies embarked on the journey of recovery, the economic transformations brought forth both opportunities and challenges.

The resilience of small businesses, a narrative of survival during the Omicron era, faced ongoing challenges in the aftermath. The economic disruptions, coupled with changes in consumer behavior and preferences, prompted local enterprises to adapt, innovate, and find new avenues for growth. The process of rebuilding and sustaining local economies became a collective endeavor that required support from communities and policymakers alike.

The gig economy, having played a crucial role in providing flexible work opportunities during the pandemic, underwent scrutiny and transformation. The conversations about workers' rights, job security, and the challenges faced by gig workers gained prominence. The need for a balanced approach that embraced the flexibility of gig work while ensuring fair labor practices became a focal point in discussions about the future of employment.

Global inequalities, magnified by the disparities in access to vaccines and resources during the pandemic, remained central considerations. The uneven distribution of economic recovery, the challenges faced by developing nations, and the imperative of addressing systemic inequities highlighted the interconnectedness of global well-being. The pursuit of a more inclusive and equitable economic framework became an integral component of the ongoing narrative.

Remote work, having become a defining feature of the Omicron era, prompted reflections on the future of work dynamics. Organizations grappled with decisions about the permanence of remote work, the balance between virtual and in-person collaboration, and the implications for employee well-being. The hybrid work model, a manifestation of the lessons learned during the pandemic, underwent further exploration and adaptation.

Job displacement and re-skilling emerged as significant themes in the post-Omicron economic landscape. The shifts in industries, the acceleration of digital transformation, and the evolving skill requirements prompted individuals to reconsider their career trajectories. The importance of continuous learning, adaptability, and the cultivation of a diverse skill set became guiding principles for navigating the dynamic job market.

Public Health Resilience and Preparedness

The Omicron era served as a stark reminder of the critical importance of public health resilience and preparedness. As societies confronted the ongoing challenges of the pandemic, reflections on healthcare systems, preventive measures, and global collaboration became central to the discourse on building a more robust and adaptive public health infrastructure.

Vaccination campaigns, having played a pivotal role in the fight against the Omicron variant, faced ongoing considerations. The need for booster doses, the emergence of new variants, and the imperative of global vaccine equity remained critical factors in shaping public health strategies. The understanding that vaccination was not only a response to a specific variant but a key component of long-term public health resilience guided ongoing efforts.

The role of technology in public health gained continued prominence. Contact tracing apps, telemedicine services, and digital platforms for health monitoring became integral tools for surveillance and early detection of potential outbreaks. The lessons learned from the pandemic underscored the potential of technology to enhance the efficiency and effectiveness of public health interventions.

Pandemic preparedness, once a topic

relegated to contingency plans, became a priority for policymakers and public health authorities. The imperative of developing resilient healthcare systems, ensuring the availability of essential medical supplies, and establishing rapid response mechanisms gained renewed attention. The understanding that pandemics were not isolated events but recurring challenges in the evolving landscape of global health prompted proactive measures.

The mental health dimensions of public health resilience became a focal point. The recognition that mental well-being was intertwined with overall health underscored the importance of integrating mental health support into public health strategies. The destigmatization of seeking mental health resources, the promotion of mental health awareness, and the incorporation of mental health considerations in healthcare policies became integral components of resilient public health frameworks.

Global Cooperation and Diplomacy

The challenges posed by the Omicron variant highlighted the interconnectedness of global health and the imperative of collaborative efforts on an international scale. As nations navigated the ongoing complexities of the post-Omicron landscape, the role of global cooperation and diplomacy emerged as a crucial element in shaping the collective response to challenges that transcended borders.

Vaccine diplomacy, once a term introduced during the race for vaccine distribution, continued to influence international relations. The collaborations between nations, pharmaceutical companies, and international organizations in ensuring vaccine accessibility to all underscored the recognition that a global response was essential to overcoming the challenges posed by the pandemic. The narratives of solidarity, support for vulnerable populations, and the acknowledgment of shared responsibilities resonated in the conversations about global health.

The geopolitical implications of the pandemic persisted in the aftermath of Omicron. Shifts in alliances, changes in diplomatic priorities, and the reassessment of global power dynamics became elements of a narrative that unfolded in the wake of the variant. The complex interplay between political considerations, economic interests, and public health imperatives shaped the diplomatic landscape in ways that reverberated far beyond the realm of healthcare.

International organizations, having played pivotal roles in coordinating responses to the pandemic, faced ongoing challenges in addressing global health disparities. The calls for reforming and strengthening international health institutions gained momentum. The understanding that a resilient global health architecture required collaborative, transparent, and inclusive mechanisms prompted discussions about the future of international cooperation in health.

The narratives of solidarity and support for vulnerable populations continued to shape global responses to humanitarian crises. The recognition that the challenges faced by one nation had implications for the collective well-being of humanity underscored the interconnectedness of global destinies. The pursuit of a more compassionate and collaborative approach to global challenges became a guiding principle in diplomatic conversations.

Cultural Shifts and Social Narratives

The cultural shifts brought about by the Omicron era continued to shape social narratives in the post-variant world. From changes in individual behaviors to transformations in societal norms, the evolution of cultural perspectives became a dynamic and ongoing aspect of the human experience.

The normalization of remote work, once an adaptation to pandemic constraints, prompted reconsiderations of work-life balance. Individuals, having experienced the flexibility of remote work, sought new ways to integrate professional responsibilities with personal pursuits. The blurring of traditional boundaries between work and leisure became a topic of reflection and adaptation.

The reevaluation of social norms surrounding health and hygiene persisted. Practices such as mask-wearing, hand hygiene, and physical distancing, once emblematic of pandemic precautions, found places in cultural routines. The ongoing awareness of health considerations in daily life prompted discussions about the lasting impact of the pandemic on societal attitudes toward well-being.

The reshaping of public spaces, from the design of urban environments to the configuration of commercial establishments, continued to reflect the adaptations prompted by the Omicron era. The emphasis on open spaces, outdoor activities, and considerations for safety in shared environments became integral components of cultural shifts in the post-variant landscape. The conversations about creating spaces that fostered community well-being, connectivity, and resilience gained momentum.

The role of technology in shaping cultural interactions remained central. Virtual events, online communities, and digital platforms continued to be conduits for connection and shared experiences. The understanding that technology could bridge distances, facilitate collaboration, and provide avenues for cultural expression prompted ongoing explorations of the digital landscape as an integral part of cultural narratives.

The impact on interpersonal relationships became a poignant theme in the evolving cultural landscape. The experiences of isolation, the reevaluation of priorities, and the acknowledgment of the importance of social connections prompted reflections on the nature of human relationships. The pursuit of meaningful connections, empathy, and understanding became guiding principles in the narratives of human interactions.

The cultural expressions of resilience, from artistic creations to community initiatives, continued to influence the stories told in the post-Omicron world. The recognition that culture was not only a reflection of societal experiences but also a driver of resilience and adaptation prompted ongoing explorations of the role of cultural narratives in shaping the collective human story.

Environmental Considerations and Sustainable Practices

The Omicron era prompted reflections on the intricate relationship between human activities, environmental health, and the imperative of sustainable practices. As societies faced the ongoing challenges of the post-variant world, the narratives of environmental considerations and sustainability unfolded as crucial components of the evolving human story.

The awareness of environmental impact persisted as a guiding principle in decision-making. From individual choices to corporate strategies, the recognition that actions had consequences for the planet prompted ongoing conversations about sustainable practices. The pursuit of a balance between human activities and ecological well-being became a central theme in the narratives of environmental considerations.

Renewable energy and green technologies gained continued attention in the post-Omicron landscape. The imperative of transitioning toward sustainable energy sources, reducing carbon emissions, and embracing eco-friendly technologies became integral components of societal discussions. The understanding that innovations in energy and technology were not only necessary for environmental health but also drivers of economic growth shaped the narratives of sustainable development.

The impact of the pandemic on biodiversity conservation became an ongoing consideration. The recognition that disruptions to ecosystems, whether through human activities or disease outbreaks, had far-reaching conse-quences for the planet underscored the interconnectedness of environmental health and human well-being. The narratives of conservation, restoration, and the coexistence of human activities with natural ecosystems became central themes in the ongoing story of environmental stewardship.

Urban planning and development faced ongoing transformations in the pursuit of sustainable practices. The design of cities, infrastructure projects, and public spaces incorporated principles of green architecture, eco-friendly transportation, and the preservation of natural habitats. The understanding that resilient urban environments were those that prioritized the well-being of both inhabitants and the planet shaped ongoing discussions about the future of cities.

Consumer behaviors underwent continued shifts toward sustainability. The choices individuals made in terms of consumption, waste reduction, and support for eco-friendly products became expressions of environmental consciousness. The narratives of conscious consumerism, circular economies, and ethical practices in business gained prominence as individuals sought ways to align their lifestyles with sustainable values.

Coping with Uncertainties and Navigating the Unknown

The uncertainties that defined the Omicron era persisted as enduring elements of the post-variant landscape. From the unpredictable nature of the virus to the complex societal transformations, individuals and communities grappled with the ongoing challenges of navigating the unknown.

The evolving nature of the virus and the emergence of new variants prompted ongoing considerations for public health measures. The adaptability of societies, the resilience of healthcare systems, and the collective commitment to protecting vulnerable populations remained essential components of the ongoing response to uncertainties in the epidemiological landscape.

The narratives of personal resilience continued to unfold as individuals faced uncertainties in various aspects of life. Career trajectories, educational pursuits, and long-term planning became arenas where adaptability, creativity, and the capacity to navigate ambiguity played crucial roles. The understanding that flexibility and a willingness to embrace change were essential qualities in navigating the unknown shaped individual stories of resilience.

The geopolitical landscape, marked by evolving global dynamics, continued to pose uncertainties. Diplomatic relationships, economic alliances, and geopolitical tensions remained fluid in the post-Omicron world. The complexities of navigating a world reshaped by both the pandemic and geopolitical shifts prompted ongoing dialogues about the role of nations in fostering stability, cooperation, and global well-being.

The social fabric, having undergone transformations during the Omicron era, continued to adapt to new norms and expectations. The considerations surrounding social interactions, cultural events, and communal gatherings remained subject to ongoing evaluations of safety, well-being, and the evolving understanding of societal responsibilities. The narratives of resilience in the face of social uncertainties became integral components of the collective human story.

The role of technology in shaping the future of human experiences remained a source of both promise and uncertainty. Advances in artificial intelligence, the integration of technology in daily life, and the ethical considerations surrounding technological innovations prompted ongoing discussions about the impact of the digital landscape on the human experience. The narratives of adaptation to technological changes and the pursuit of a balanced relationship between humanity and technology became ongoing themes in societal conversations.

Global efforts to address climate change and environmental degradation faced ongoing challenges. The uncertainties surrounding the pace of environmental transformations, the effectiveness of mitigation strategies, and the commitment of nations to sustainable practices shaped the ongoing narrative of environmental stewardship. The recognition that the planet faced a future marked by both challenges and opportunities prompted discussions about the role of individuals, communities, and nations in building a resilient and sustainable world.

As individuals and communities navigated the uncertainties that persisted in the post-Omicron era, the importance of resilience, adaptability, and a shared commitment to collective well-being became guiding principles. The narratives of triumphs over adversity, the ongoing challenges faced by societies, and the human capacity to confront the unknown with courage and determination continued to shape the evolving human story.

Embracing the Unwritten Chapters

In the chapters that follow, the human journey unfolds with its complexities, triumphs, and ongoing adaptations. The unwritten chapters of the post-Omicron world invite individuals and communities to contribute their stories to the collective narrative of human resilience. From the realms of health and economics to diplomacy, culture, and the environment, each facet of the human experience becomes a brushstroke in the canvas of a future shaped by the lessons learned during the pandemic.

The narratives of hope, renewal, and resilience serve as guiding beacons as humanity embarks on the journey of embracing the unwritten chapters. The challenges that remain, the triumphs yet to be celebrated, and the ongoing evolution of societal norms beckon individuals to contribute their voices, experiences, and visions for a future that reflects the values of compassion, collaboration, and sustainable coexistence.

In the unwritten chapters, individuals find opportunities to redefine personal and collective narratives. The stories of innovation, community building, and the pursuit of equity become threads that weave the fabric of a future where the human spirit continues to demonstrate its indomitable strength. The embrace of uncertainties becomes a testament to the enduring capacity of humanity to adapt, learn, and create pathways toward a better world.

As we venture into the unwritten chapters, the human story becomes a canvas where each person contributes a stroke of resilience, a shade of adaptation, and a hue of hope. The challenges that emerge, the societal transformations that unfold, and the triumphs that mark the journey become part of a narrative that transcends borders, cultures, and individual experiences. In the unwritten chapters, the human spirit finds space to reimagine, recreate, and contribute to a shared destiny where the echoes of the Omicron era become notes in a symphony of human perseverance.

The Essence of Human Connection

In the intricate fabric of the post-Omicron world, the theme of human connection emerges as a defining thread. As societies navigate the challenges and triumphs of the evolving landscape, the narratives of relationships, community bonds, and shared humanity become central elements in the human story. In this chapter, we unravel the layers of the tapestry of human connection, exploring the nuances of interpersonal relationships, community resilience, and the enduring capacity of humans to find strength in unity.

Rediscovering the Beauty of Face-to-Face Connections

The embrace of face-to-face interactions in the post-Omicron era becomes a poignant chapter in the story of human connection. The return to physical gatherings, the warmth of shared spaces, and the joy of in-person conversations mark a renaissance in the way individuals experience one another. The nuanced expressions, the subtle cues of body language, and the shared energy of being present in the same physical space become cherished aspects of human connection.

The impact of physical distancing measures during the pandemic prompted a reevaluation of the significance of proximity in human relationships. The simple acts of a handshake, a hug, or the shared experience of a meal gain newfound importance in the post-variant world. Individuals savor the sensory richness of direct interactions, rediscovering the beauty of genuine, unfiltered human connections.

As communities rekindle the flame of shared experiences, from family gatherings to community events, the communal spirit takes center stage. The laughter, the tears, and the collective celebration of milestones become not just moments but expressions of the human need for connection. The shared narratives of resilience, adapted traditions, and the collective joy of reunions become chapters in the evolving story of human relationships.

Navigating the Complexities of Social Reintegration

The process of social reintegration, though marked by joyous reunions, unfolds with its complexities. Individuals, having adapted to the nuances of virtual interactions, find themselves navigating the intricacies of face-to-face relationships in the post-Omicron world. The journey involves a delicate balance between the comfort of solitude and the enriching dynamics of communal connections.

Social anxiety, a companion through the uncertainties of the pandemic, finds resonance in the process of social reintegration. The apprehension about reestablishing connections, the uncertainties about societal norms, and the evolving landscape of social interactions become elements of the human experience. The narratives of individuals navigating the complexities of reconnecting with friends, family, and communities weave into the broader tapestry of human connection.

The recalibration of social norms prompts ongoing conversations about boundaries, consent, and the evolving expectations in interpersonal relationships. Individuals engage in dialogues about personal comfort levels, the nuances of consent in physical interactions, and the mutual understanding required in the delicate dance of social reintegration. The narratives of open communication, empathy, and the collective commitment to creating inclusive spaces become integral components of the evolving social landscape.

The role of technology in social reintegration remains significant. Virtual connections, cultivated during the pandemic, coexist with face-to-face interactions, offering individuals a spectrum of choices in how they connect with others. The understanding that technology can complement and enhance, rather than replace, human connections becomes a guiding principle in the ongoing exploration of social dynamics.

Community Resilience: Bonds that Withstand Challenges

The resilience of communities becomes a powerful testament to the strength of human connection. From the local neighborhoods to global networks, the bonds forged during the challenges of the Omicron era continue to shape the collective resilience of communities. The narratives of mutual support, shared resources, and the recognition of interconnected destinies become chapters in the story of communities navigating uncertainties.

Local communities, having weathered the storms of the pandemic, emerge as crucibles of resilience. The support networks established during the Omicron era, from mutual aid groups to community initiatives, lay the foundation for ongoing collaborations. The understanding that the well-being of each individual is intertwined with the well-being of the community becomes a guiding principle in the narratives of localized resilience.

The importance of inclusivity in community resilience gains prominence. The narratives of communities that prioritize the needs of vulnerable populations, embrace diversity, and foster a sense of belonging become exemplars of the transformative power of human connection. The shared commitment to leaving no one behind, especially in times of crisis, becomes a rallying cry for communities building resilience in the post-Omicron world.

Global networks, interconnected by shared experiences, continue to evolve in the aftermath of the variant. The lessons learned from international collaborations, the recognition of the value of shared knowledge, and the imperative of global solidarity shape ongoing dialogues about the interconnected destinies of nations. The narratives of nations supporting one another, sharing resources, and collectively addressing global challenges become integral components of the evolving story of human connection on a global scale.

The Impact of Interpersonal Relationships on Mental Well-being

The profound impact of interpersonal relationships on mental well-being takes center stage in the post-Omicron narrative. As individuals navigate the complexities of the human experience, from the joys of connection to the challenges of social dynamics, the stories of mental health and resilience unfold in the context of relationships.

The support systems established during the Omicron era continue to play a crucial role in mental well-being. The narratives of friends checking in on one another, families creating spaces for open conversations, and communities fostering environments of understanding become testimonials to the healing power of human connection. The importance of nurturing relationships as pillars of mental health resilience becomes a central theme in the evolving human story.

Loneliness, a shadow that loomed large during periods of isolation, prompts ongoing reflections on the role of relationships in combating social isolation. The narratives of individuals reaching out, forging new connections, and embracing the richness of social bonds become beacons of hope for those grappling with the emotional toll of loneliness. The recognition that human connections serve as antidotes to isolation underscores the significance of relationships in the pursuit of mental well-being.

The complexities of interpersonal dynamics, from familial relationships to friendships and romantic connections, become themes in the stories of individuals navigating the post-Omicron world. The narratives of forgiveness, understanding, and the resilience required in the face of relational challenges become integral components of the human experience. The acknowledgment that the tapestry of human connection is woven with threads of imperfection adds depth to the ongoing exploration of relationships.

Cultural Connections: Celebrating Diversity and Shared Humanity

Cultural connections, celebrated for their richness and diversity, become vibrant threads in the tapestry of human connection. The post-Omicron era invites individuals and communities to explore the intersections of cultures, embrace diversity, and find unity in the shared elements of the human experience. The narratives of cultural connections transcend borders, fostering understanding and appreciation for the myriad ways people express their identities.

The renaissance of cultural events, festivals, and celebrations marks a chapter of renewal in the post-variant world. Communities, having adapted traditions during the challenges of the pandemic, find joy in the resumption

of cultural expressions. The narratives of shared festivities, the vibrancy of cultural exchanges, and the collective pride in diverse heritage become integral components of the evolving cultural landscape.

Cultural connections serve as bridges between communities, fostering a sense of shared humanity. The narratives of individuals exploring cultures different from their own, engaging in cross-cultural dialogues, and embracing the beauty of diversity become testimonials to the capacity of human connection to transcend cultural boundaries. The shared stories of individuals finding common ground, despite cultural differences, underscore the universal desire for connection and understanding.

The role of technology in fostering cultural connections gains continued significance. Virtual platforms, digital spaces, and online communities become avenues for individuals to engage with diverse cultures, share experiences, and celebrate the richness of global diversity. The understanding that technology can be a tool for cultural exchange and mutual understanding becomes a guiding principle in the ongoing exploration of cultural connections.

Challenges in the Tapestry: Navigating Disconnections and Strained Relationships

Amidst the celebration of human connection, the tapestry reveals threads of challenges and disconnections. The complexities of interpersonal relationships, the strains of social dynamics, and the evolving societal norms prompt ongoing reflections on the fragility of human connections. The narratives of individuals navigating relational challenges, experiencing disconnections, and grappling with the complexities of strained relationships become integral components of the human story.

The impact of prolonged isolation on social skills and relational dynamics becomes a theme in the post-Omicron world. Individuals, having adapted to virtual interactions, find themselves navigating the intricacies of face-to-face communication. The narratives of individuals experiencing social awkwardness, miscommunications, and the challenges of reconnecting with others become reflections on the evolving nature of human connections.

Relational challenges within families, marked by the pressures of the pandemic, continue to shape individual narratives. The complexities of balancing familial responsibilities, the strains of caregiving, and the evolving roles within family structures prompt ongoing conversations about the dynamics of family relationships. The narratives of individuals seeking support, setting boundaries, and navigating familial expectations become stories of resilience in the face of familial challenges.

Friendships, tested by the uncertainties of the pandemic, undergo transformations in the post-Omicron era. The narratives of individuals renegotiating the dynamics of friendships, addressing conflicts, and navigating changes in social circles become integral components of the evolving human story. The recognition that friendships, like all relationships, require effort, understanding, and adaptability becomes a guiding principle in the ongoing exploration of social connections.

The impact of societal changes on romantic relationships prompts ongoing considerations. The narratives of individuals navigating the complexities of dating, reevaluating priorities in partnerships, and addressing the challenges of intimacy in the post-variant world become reflections on the evolving landscape of romantic connections. The shared stories of individuals finding resilience, adapting to relational changes, and redefining the meaning of connection in romantic relationships become integral components of the evolving human narrative.

Technology and the Evolution of Human Connection

The role of technology in shaping human connection undergoes continued exploration in the post-Omicron world. From the innovations that facilitated virtual connections during the pandemic to the ongoing integration of technology into daily life, the narratives of human-technology interactions become integral components of the evolving human story.

Virtual connections, once a lifeline during periods of isolation, continue to coexist with face-to-face interactions. The narratives of individuals maintaining meaningful relationships through virtual platforms, connecting with loved ones across distances, and participating in online communities become stories of the adaptability and resilience of human connections. The understanding that technology serves as a bridge, connecting individuals in diverse corners of the world, becomes a central theme in the exploration of virtual connections.

The impact of technology on the dynamics of communication and social interactions prompts ongoing considerations. The narratives of individuals navigating the challenges of digital communication, addressing the complexities of online relationships, and finding balance in the use of technology become reflections on the evolving nature of human connections. The shared stories of individuals setting boundaries, fostering meaningful connections in digital spaces, and leveraging technology as a tool for positive interactions become integral components of the ongoing exploration of technology and human connection.

The ethical considerations surrounding technology and privacy become themes in the evolving human narrative. The narratives of individuals grappling with concerns about data security, the impact of social media on mental well-being, and the ethical use of emerging technologies become reflections on the responsibilities inherent in the intersection of technology and human connection. The understanding that conscious choices in digital interactions contribute to the cultivation of healthy and meaningful connections becomes a guiding principle in the ongoing exploration of technology in the post-Omicron world.

The Future of Human Connection: A Collective Journey

As we navigate the intricate tapestry of human connection in the post-Omicron world, the future unfolds as a collective journey. The narratives of individuals, communities, and cultures intertwine, creating a story that transcends individual experiences. From the celebrations of shared moments to the challenges of strained relationships, each thread in the tapestry contributes to the rich narrative of human connection.

The essence of human connection lies in the shared experiences, the empathy that bridges differences, and the collective commitment to building a world where everyone feels seen, heard, and valued. The ongoing exploration of human connection in the post-Omicron era becomes an invitation for individuals to contribute their stories, experiences, and perspectives to the evolving human narrative.

The Dynamic Rhythms of Change

In the post-Omicron landscape, the dance of cultural shifts takes center stage, revealing the intricate choreography of evolving societal norms and values. As communities navigate the echoes of the pandemic, the narratives of change unfold in the ways people interact, celebrate, and shape the collective identity. In this chapter, we delve into the dynamic rhythms of cultural shifts, exploring the nuances of transformation in social interactions, gatherings, and the fabric of human connection.

The Unfolding Canvas of Societal Norms

The canvas of societal norms undergoes a nuanced transformation in the post-Omicron era, reflecting the evolving values and perspectives of communities. As individuals and societies emerge from the shadows of the pandemic, the narratives of societal norms become chapters in the ongoing story of adaptation, resilience, and the pursuit of a new equilibrium.

One prominent theme is the reevaluation of work-life balance. The experiences of remote work during the pandemic prompt ongoing reflections on the traditional structures of work. Individuals, having tasted the flexibility of remote arrangements, seek a balance that allows them to integrate professional responsibilities with personal pursuits. The narratives of individuals negotiating flexible work hours, reimagining office spaces, and prioritizing well-being become brushstrokes on the canvas of reshaped societal norms.

The dynamics of gender roles undergo scrutiny in the post-Omicron landscape. The pandemic, with its disruptions to established routines, prompts conversations about caregiving responsibilities, domestic partnerships, and the evolving expectations within families. The narratives of individuals challenging gender stereotypes, advocating for equality, and fostering environments that embrace diverse expressions of gender roles become integral components of the evolving societal narrative.

The recalibration of cultural attitudes toward mental health becomes a central theme. The collective experiences of navigating the uncertainties and stresses of the pandemic prompt a reevaluation of the stigma surrounding mental well-being. The narratives of individuals openly discussing mental health, seeking support, and fostering environments that prioritize emotional well-being become testimonials to the changing tides of societal attitudes toward mental health.

Generational shifts contribute to the evolving tapestry of societal norms. The experiences of younger generations, marked by the challenges of the pandemic, shape their perspectives on issues such as education, career choices, and social responsibility. The narratives of younger individuals advocating for systemic change, reimagining traditional institutions, and challenging established norms become integral components of the broader societal dialogue.

The inclusion of diverse voices becomes a driving force in the reshaping of societal norms. The narratives of marginalized communities, previously relegated to the periphery, gain prominence as individuals demand equity, representation, and the acknowledgment of the rich tapestry of human experiences. The understanding that societal norms must be inclusive, respectful of diversity, and attentive to historically marginalized perspectives becomes a guiding principle in the ongoing cultural shifts.

Transformations in Social Interactions: From Digital to Physical Connections

The dynamics of social interactions undergo a profound transformation in the post-Omicron world, transitioning from the virtual spaces that defined the pandemic to a renewed emphasis on face-to-face connections. The narratives of individuals navigating this shift reveal the complexities, joys, and challenges of recalibrating the ways people engage with one another.

Virtual connections, once a lifeline during periods of isolation, coexist with face-to-face interactions. The narratives of individuals maintaining meaningful relationships through virtual platforms, connecting with loved ones across distances, and participating in online communities become stories of adaptability and resilience. The understanding that technology can be a bridge, connecting individuals in diverse corners of the world, becomes a central theme in the exploration of social interactions.

The resurgence of face-to-face interactions brings both joy and challenges. Individuals, having adapted to the nuances of virtual conversations, find themselves navigating the intricacies of in-person communication. The narratives of individuals experiencing social awkwardness, miscommunications, and the challenges of reconnecting with others become reflections on the evolving nature of human connections.

The complexities of social reintegration prompt ongoing considerations about boundaries, consent, and the evolving expectations in interpersonal relationships. The narratives of individuals engaging in open communication, expressing personal comfort levels, and fostering mutual understanding become integral components of the evolving social landscape. The understanding that navigating social interactions requires collective awareness, empathy, and respect for individual choices becomes a guiding principle in the exploration of transformed social dynamics.

The role of technology in enhancing physical interactions gains continued significance. From the use of contactless technologies in public spaces to the integration of digital tools in event planning, technology becomes a facilitator of seamless and safe face-to-face interactions. The narratives of individuals embracing technological innovations to enhance the quality of physical connections underscore the potential of technology as a tool for positive social interactions.

The revitalization of community gatherings becomes a vibrant chapter in the story of transformed social interactions. From local events to global festivals, communities rediscover the joy of shared experiences. The narratives of individuals participating in cultural celebrations, communal gatherings, and collective expressions of joy become integral components of the evolving human story. The understanding that shared moments of celebration contribute to the vibrancy of social connections becomes a central theme in the exploration of transformed social interactions.

Celebrating Diversity: The Evolution of Cultural Expressions

Cultural expressions undergo a renaissance in the post-Omicron era, becoming dynamic reflections of the evolving human experience. From changes in artistic creations to the reimagining of communal spaces, the narratives of cultural shifts reveal the ways in which communities celebrate diversity, express resilience, and shape the cultural identity of the post-variant world.

The arts, having served as sources of solace and inspiration during the pandemic, continue to evolve in the post-Omicron landscape. The narratives of artists exploring new themes, experimenting with diverse mediums, and contributing to the collective healing through their creations become integral components of the evolving cultural tapestry. The understanding that art serves as a mirror to societal experiences and a catalyst for cultural dialogue becomes a guiding principle in the exploration of transformed cultural expressions.

Cultural events, festivals, and celebrations mark a chapter of renewal in the post-variant world. Communities, having adapted traditions during the challenges of the pandemic, find joy in the resumption of cultural expressions. The narratives of shared festivities, the vibrancy of cultural exchanges, and the collective pride in diverse heritage become integral components of the evolving cultural landscape. The understanding that cultural celebrations contribute to the sense of belonging, foster community resilience, and connect individuals across diverse backgrounds becomes a central theme in the exploration of transformed cultural expressions.

The reshaping of public spaces becomes a reflection of cultural shifts. Urban environments, once defined by bustling crowds and shared spaces, undergo transformations to accommodate the evolving needs of communities. The narratives of individuals participating in the design of public spaces, advocating for inclusive urban planning, and fostering environments that prioritize cultural vibrancy become testimonials to the transformative power of community engagement in

shaping cultural expressions.

Digital platforms continue to play a central role in cultural connections. Virtual events, online communities, and digital collaborations become conduits for cultural exchange and shared experiences. The narratives of individuals leveraging technology to amplify cultural voices, connect with global audiences, and create digital spaces that celebrate diversity become integral components of the evolving cultural narrative. The understanding that technology can be a tool for democratizing cultural expressions and fostering global dialogue becomes a guiding principle in the exploration of transformed cultural landscapes.

The Impact on Traditions and Rituals: Navigating Change with Reverence

Traditions and rituals, woven into the fabric of cultural identities, undergo a delicate transformation in the post-Omicron era. The narratives of individuals navigating changes in longstanding practices, reevaluating the significance of rituals, and adapting traditions to the evolving cultural landscape reveal the ways in which communities navigate the dance between continuity and change.

The celebration of major life events takes on new dimensions. Weddings, birthdays, and other milestones become occasions for reflection on the evolving meaning of these rituals. The narratives of individuals reimagining traditional ceremonies, incorporating modern elements, and embracing a sense of individuality in their celebrations become integral components of the evolving human story. The understanding that rituals can be meaningful expressions of cultural identity while also evolving to reflect contemporary values becomes a central theme in the exploration of transformed traditions.

Religious practices undergo adaptations in response to the challenges of the pandemic. The narratives of individuals participating in virtual religious services, exploring new modes of spiritual connection, and fostering inclusive spaces for diverse beliefs become testimonials to the resilience of faith communities. The understanding that spirituality can transcend physical spaces and find expression in innovative forms becomes a guiding principle in the exploration of transformed religious practices.

Ceremonies of remembrance and mourning gain added significance in the post-Omicron landscape. The narratives of individuals navigating the complexities of grief, finding solace in communal rituals, and creating spaces for collective healing become integral components of the evolving human story. The understanding that traditions surrounding loss and remembrance play a crucial role in the healing process becomes a central theme in the exploration of transformed rituals.

Generational perspectives contribute to the evolving narrative of traditions and rituals. The experiences of younger generations, influenced by the challenges of the pandemic, prompt reflections on the relevance and meaning of longstanding practices. The narratives of individuals reinterpreting traditions, infusing new elements into rituals, and contributing to the ongoing evolution of cultural practices become integral components of the broader dialogue about the role of traditions in the post-Omicron world.

Challenges and Opportunities in Cultural Shifts

Amidst the celebrations of cultural shifts, the tapestry reveals threads of challenges and opportunities. The complexities of navigating societal changes, the strains on cultural expressions, and the evolving dynamics of human connections prompt ongoing reflections on the fragility and resilience of cultural identities. The narratives of individuals grappling with the uncertainties of change, addressing cultural disconnections, and fostering environments that celebrate diversity become integral components of the evolving human story.

The impact of global influences on local cultures prompts ongoing con-siderations. The narratives of individuals navigating the complexities of cultural globalization, seeking to preserve cultural authenticity, and fostering environments that value both local and global identities become reflections on the challenges and opportunities inherent in the interconnected world. The understanding that cultural shifts require intentional efforts to balance preservation and adaptation becomes a guiding principle in the exploration of transformed cultural landscapes.

The role of education in shaping cultural awareness gains prominence. The narratives of individuals advocating for inclusive curricula, fostering cultural literacy, and creating spaces for intercultural dialogue become testimonials to the transformative power of education in navigating cultural shifts. The understanding that education plays a crucial role in shaping the perspectives of future generations and fostering cultural understanding becomes a central theme in the exploration of transformed cultural identities.

The impact of economic disparities on cultural expressions becomes a theme in the evolving narrative. The narratives of individuals navigating the challenges of economic constraints, advocating for equitable access to cultural resources, and fostering environments that prioritize cultural vibrancy irrespective of socio-economic backgrounds become reflections on the intersection of culture and economic realities. The understanding that cultural shifts must address issues of accessibility, representation, and inclusivity becomes a guiding principle in the exploration of transformed cultural landscapes.

The complexities of balancing tradition with progress prompt ongoing dialogues. The narratives of individuals negotiating the tensions between preserving cultural heritage and embracing innovation become integral components of the broader conversation about cultural shifts. The understanding that cultural resilience requires a dynamic interplay between tradition and progress becomes a central theme in the exploration of transformed cultural identities.

The Future of Cultural Shifts: A Living Tapestry

As we navigate the dance of cultural shifts in the post-Omicron world, the future emerges as a living tapestry shaped by the stories, experiences, and aspirations of individuals and communities. From the celebrations of diverse cultural expressions to the challenges of preserving traditions, each thread in the tapestry contributes to the rich narrative of cultural shifts.

The essence of cultural shifts lies in the recognition that societies are dynamic, ever-evolving entities. The ongoing exploration of cultural shifts in the post-Omicron era becomes an invitation for individuals to contribute their stories, experiences, and perspectives to the evolving human narrative. As communities engage in dialogues about the meaning of cultural identity, the role of traditions, and the celebration of diversity, the tapestry becomes a testament to the beauty, resilience, and transformative power of cultural shifts in the post-Omicron world.

A Symphony of Resilience

In the intricate symphony of human existence, the melody of resilience echoes through the post-Omicron world. As communities navigate the aftermath of the variant, the narratives of resilience become the heartbeat of the evolving human story. In this chapter, we explore the nuances of this symphony, delving into the stories of individuals, communities, and societies finding strength in the face of challenges, adapting to uncertainties, and contributing to the collective resilience that shapes the post-variant era.

Individual Resilience: Narratives of Personal Triumphs

At the heart of the symphony are the individual stories of resilience, where triumphs over adversity become notes in the melody of human strength. The narratives of individuals navigating the complexities of the post-Omicron landscape reveal the myriad ways in which personal resilience manifests.

The journey of health and recovery takes center stage. The narratives of individuals who faced the challenges of illness, emerged from the shadows of the variant, and embarked on the path of recovery become testimonials to the indomitable human spirit. The stories of physical strength, mental fortitude, and the emotional resilience required in the face of health uncertainties contribute vibrant notes to the symphony of individual resilience.

The pursuit of personal growth and self-discovery becomes a recurring theme. Individuals, having weathered the storms of the pandemic, share narratives of reevaluating priorities, embracing new passions, and finding purpose in the midst of challenges. The understanding that resilience extends beyond survival to the transformative power of personal growth becomes a guiding principle in the exploration of individual resilience.

Economic resilience takes on added significance in the post-Omicron era. The narratives of individuals navigating the complexities of economic uncertainties, adapting to changes in employment landscapes, and finding innovative ways to sustain livelihoods become integral components of the evolving human story. The stories of entrepreneurship, adaptability, and the pursuit of financial well-being underscore the economic resilience that resonates in the symphony of human strength.

The complexities of mental health resilience emerge as central themes. Individuals share narratives of navigating anxiety, facing periods of isolation, and finding pathways to emotional well-being. The stories of seeking therapy, cultivating mindfulness practices, and fostering environments that prioritize mental health contribute essential notes to the symphony of individual resilience. The understanding that mental well-being is a crucial aspect of personal resilience becomes a central theme in the exploration of individual stories.

The pursuit of meaningful connections becomes a source of resilience for many. The narratives of individuals forging new relationships, reconnecting with loved ones, and creating supportive social networks underscore the importance of human connections in the symphony of resilience. The stories of individuals navigating the complexities of social dynamics, finding solace in shared experiences, and contributing to communal well-being become integral components of the evolving human narrative.

Community Resilience: Threads of Collective Strength

The symphony of resilience extends beyond individual stories to encompass the collective strength of communities. Local neighborhoods, global networks, and diverse communities contribute threads to the tapestry of community resilience, revealing the power of shared experiences, mutual support, and the collaborative pursuit of well-being.

Mutual aid initiatives become beacons of community resilience. The narratives of individuals coming together to support vulnerable members of the community, share resources, and foster a sense of collective responsibility become integral components of the evolving human story. The stories of neighbors checking in on one another, community leaders organizing support networks, and the recognition that the well-being of each individual is interconnected with the well-being of the community resonate in the symphony of community resilience.

The role of cultural organizations in fostering resilience gains prominence. The narratives of communities celebrating cultural expressions, supporting local artists, and creating spaces for collective healing become integral components of the evolving cultural landscape. The stories of cultural institutions adapting to challenges, embracing digital platforms, and contributing to the vibrancy of community life underscore the role of cultural resilience in the symphony of community strength.

Global collaborations become a testament to the interconnected destinies of nations. The narratives of international cooperation, the sharing of resources, and the collective response to global challenges become integral components of the evolving geopolitical landscape. The stories of nations supporting one another, engaging in diplomatic dialogues, and recognizing the shared vulnerabilities and opportunities in the post-Omicron world contribute to the symphony of global resilience.

Educational institutions play a crucial role in community resilience. The narratives of schools adapting to new modes of learning, educators fostering environments of understanding and support, and students navigating the challenges of education in the post-Omicron era become integral components of the evolving educational narrative. The stories of resilience in the face of educational disruptions, the pursuit of innovative teaching methods, and the commitment to nurturing the next generation of resilient individuals contribute to the symphony of community strength.

Innovations and Adaptations: Orchestrating Change

The symphony of resilience is marked by the innovative notes of adaptation, where individuals and communities orchestrate change in response to the challenges of the post-Omicron world. The narratives of innovative solutions, adaptive strategies, and transformative initiatives reveal the ways in which resilience translates into actions that shape the future.

Technological innovations become instrumental in the symphony of re-silience. The narratives of individuals and organizations leveraging tech-nology to address challenges, connect communities, and foster innovation contribute to the evolving digital landscape. The stories of technological adaptations in healthcare, education, and social interactions underscore the transformative power of innovation in the symphony of resilience.

Entrepreneurial resilience becomes a driving force for economic adaptation. The narratives of individuals starting new businesses, embracing digital entrepreneurship, and finding innovative solutions to economic challenges become integral components of the evolving economic narrative. The stories of small businesses pivoting to meet changing demands, entrepreneurs navigating uncertainties, and communities supporting local economies contribute to the symphony of economic resilience.

Environmental resilience takes on added significance. The narratives of individuals and communities prioritizing sustainable practices, engaging in conservation efforts, and addressing climate change become integral compo-nents of the evolving environmental narrative. The stories of innovations in renewable energy, sustainable agriculture, and the recognition of the interconnectedness of environmental well-being with human well-being resonate in the symphony of resilience.

The transformation of healthcare systems becomes a key theme. The narratives of individuals working in healthcare, adapting to evolving medical landscapes, and contributing to public health initiatives become integral components of the evolving healthcare narrative. The stories of healthcare professionals navigating challenges, implementing telemedicine solutions, and advocating for inclusive healthcare practices contribute to the symphony of resilience in the face of health uncertainties.

Cultural adaptations contribute to the vibrancy of the symphony. The narratives of artists exploring new mediums, cultural institutions embracing digital expressions, and communities reimagining traditional practices become integral components of the evolving cultural landscape. The stories of resilience in the face of cultural challenges, the celebration of diverse expressions, and the commitment to preserving cultural heritage contribute to the symphony of cultural strength.

The Social Fabric: Weaving Resilient Communities

At the core of the symphony of resilience is the intricate weaving of the social fabric, where communities come together to support, uplift, and celebrate the human spirit. The narratives of social resilience reveal the ways in which individuals contribute to the collective strength that defines the post-Omicron era.

The importance of empathy becomes a recurring theme. The narratives of individuals demonstrating compassion, understanding, and a willingness to listen to one another contribute to the evolving social landscape. The stories of empathy in action, whether in personal relationships, community initiatives, or global collaborations, become integral components of the symphony of social resilience.

Inclusive practices become guiding principles in the symphony of resilience

. The narratives of individuals advocating for inclusivity, challenging systemic inequalities, and fostering environments that value diversity become integral components of the evolving social narrative. The stories of inclusivity in education, employment, and community spaces underscore the transformative power of social resilience in building a more equitable post-Omicron world.

Collective healing becomes a central theme in the symphony of resilience. The narratives of individuals and communities creating spaces for shared grief, supporting one another in times of loss, and fostering environments of emotional well-being become integral components of the evolving human story. The stories of collective healing in the face of trauma, uncertainty, and societal challenges contribute to the symphony of social strength.

The role of education in shaping resilient communities gains prominence. The narratives of schools fostering environments of understanding, empathy, and support become integral components of the evolving educational narrative. The stories of educators guiding students through the complexities of the post-Omicron world, students engaging in dialogue about societal challenges, and educational institutions becoming hubs for social awareness contribute to the symphony of social resilience.

Challenges and Opportunities in the Symphony of Resilience

Amidst the harmony of resilience, challenges and opportunities emerge as integral components of the symphony. The complexities of navigating personal, community, and societal resilience prompt ongoing reflections on the fragility and strength of the human spirit. The narratives of individuals grappling with uncertainties, addressing systemic challenges, and fostering environments that prioritize well-being become integral components of the evolving human story.

Economic disparities remain a challenge in the symphony of resilience. The narratives of individuals navigating the impact of economic constraints, advocating for equitable opportunities, and fostering environments that prioritize economic inclusivity become reflections on the intersection of economic realities and resilience. The understanding that resilience must address issues of accessibility, representation, and economic well-being becomes a guiding principle in the exploration of economic challenges in the post-Omicron world.

Mental health disparities prompt ongoing considerations. The narratives of individuals navigating the complexities of mental health, addressing stigma, and fostering environments that prioritize emotional well-being become reflections on the challenges and opportunities inherent in the symphony of resilience. The understanding that mental health resilience requires collective efforts, empathy, and a commitment to destigmatizing mental health becomes a central theme in the exploration of mental health challenges.

Social inequalities remain a focal point in the evolving narrative of resilience. The narratives of individuals challenging systemic injustices, advocating for social equity, and fostering environments that value diversity become reflections on the challenges and opportunities in the symphony of resilience. The understanding that social resilience requires intentional efforts to address systemic inequalities and create inclusive spaces becomes a guiding principle in the exploration of social challenges in the post-Omicron world.

The complexities of global interdependence prompt ongoing dialogues. The narratives of individuals navigating the challenges of geopolitical landscapes, contributing to global collaborations, and fostering environments that prioritize international cooperation become reflections on the opportunities and challenges inherent in the symphony of resilience. The understanding that global resilience requires diplomatic efforts, mutual support, and a recognition of shared vulnerabilities becomes a central theme in the exploration of global challenges in the post-Omicron era.

The Future of Resilience: A Collective Overture

As we navigate the symphony of resilience in the post-Omicron world, the future emerges as a collective overture shaped by the stories, experiences, and aspirations of individuals and communities. From the triumphs of personal resilience to the strength of interconnected communities, each note in the symphony contributes to the rich narrative of resilience.

The essence of resilience lies in the recognition that challenges are inherent in the human experience, but so too is the capacity for adaptation, growth, and collective strength. The ongoing exploration of resilience in the post-Omicron era becomes an invitation for individuals to contribute their stories, experiences, and perspectives to the evolving human narrative. As communities engage in dialogues about the meaning of resilience, the role of collective well-being, and the importance of fostering environments that nurture the human spirit, the symphony becomes a living testament to the beauty, strength, and transformative power of resilience in the post-Omicron world.

Echoes of Hope

In the aftermath of the Omicron variant, a new chapter unfolds—one that resonates with the melody of hope. As individuals and communities navigate the complexities of the post-Omicron era, the narratives of hope become the guiding light illuminating the path forward. In this chapter, we explore the multifaceted dimensions of hope, delving into the stories of resilience, renewal, and the enduring human spirit that shape the post-variant world.

Individual Hopes: The Seeds of Personal Renewal

At the heart of the chapter on hope are the individual stories that weave a tapestry of personal renewal. Each narrative is a testament to the power of hope in transforming challenges into opportunities, setbacks into comebacks, and uncertainty into a journey of self-discovery.

The pursuit of personal goals becomes a beacon of hope. Individuals share stories of setting new aspirations, redefining success, and embracing the journey rather than fixating on destinations. The narratives of resilience in the face of setbacks, the joy of small victories, and the commitment to personal growth contribute to the evolving human story of hope.

Reconnection with passions and purpose becomes a central theme. The narratives of individuals rediscovering hobbies, reigniting creative sparks, and aligning their lives with a sense of purpose become integral components of the tapestry of hope. The stories of individuals who find fulfillment in pursuing their passions, whether artistic, philanthropic, or intellectual, resonate as notes in the melody of personal renewal.

The embrace of positive habits and well-being practices takes on added significance. Individuals share stories of cultivating mindfulness, adopting healthy lifestyles, and prioritizing self-care. The narratives of individuals navigating the complexities of mental well-being, embracing practices that contribute to emotional resilience, and fostering environments that prioritize holistic health contribute to the evolving human story of hope.

Educational aspirations and lifelong learning become sources of hope. The narratives of individuals pursuing education, upskilling, and engaging in continuous learning reveal the transformative power of knowledge. The stories of individuals navigating the challenges of education, adapting to new learning environments, and embracing the opportunities for intellectual growth become integral components of the evolving educational narrative of hope.

The pursuit of meaningful connections becomes a cornerstone of individual hope. Individuals share narratives of forging new relationships, repairing existing bonds, and contributing to the vibrancy of social connections. The stories of individuals who find solace in shared experiences, foster empathy in relationships, and contribute to the well-being of their communities resonate as essential notes in the symphony of individual hope.

Community Hopes: Collective Aspirations for Renewal

The melody of hope extends beyond individual stories to encompass the collective aspirations of communities. The narratives of community renewal, collaboration, and shared visions for a better future become integral threads in the tapestry of hope that defines the post-Omicron world.

Community-led initiatives become beacons of hope. The narratives of individuals coming together to address local challenges, foster inclusivity, and create spaces for collective well-being contribute to the evolving human story of community hope. The stories of neighbors supporting one another, grassroots organizations leading change, and communities becoming hubs for resilience resonate as powerful notes in the melody of community renewal.

Cultural celebrations and expressions mark a chapter of hope. Communities share stories of reviving traditional practices, hosting festivals, and embracing the vibrancy of cultural diversity. The narratives of individuals participating in cultural events, supporting local artists, and fostering environments that celebrate heritage contribute to the evolving cultural landscape of hope.

Environmental stewardship becomes a shared hope for communities. The narratives of individuals and groups advocating for sustainable practices, engaging in conservation efforts, and prioritizing environmental well-being contribute to the evolving environmental narrative of hope. The stories of communities fostering green initiatives, implementing eco-friendly practices, and raising awareness about the interconnectedness of human and environmental health resonate as essential notes in the melody of collective hope.

The role of education in shaping hopeful communities gains prominence. The narratives of schools fostering environments of understanding, empathy, and social responsibility become integral components of the evolving educational narrative of hope. The stories of educators guiding students through the complexities of the post-Omicron world, students engaging in dialogue about societal challenges, and educational institutions becoming hubs for social awareness contribute to the symphony of community hope.

Innovations and Transformations: A Symphony of Hopeful Change

Hope is a driving force behind innovations and transformations that shape the post-Omicron landscape. The narratives of individuals and communities orchestrating change, embracing creativity, and contributing to positive shifts in various domains become integral threads in the tapestry of hopeful change.

Technological innovations become instruments of hope. The narratives of individuals and organizations leveraging technology to address challenges, connect communities, and foster innovation contribute to the evolving digital landscape of hope. The stories of technological adaptations in healthcare, education, and social interactions underscore the transformative power of innovation in the symphony of hopeful change.

Entrepreneurial ventures become expressions of hope. The narratives of individuals starting new businesses, embracing digital entrepreneurship, and finding innovative solutions to economic challenges become integral components of the evolving economic narrative of hope. The stories of small businesses pivoting to meet changing demands, entrepreneurs navigating uncertainties, and communities supporting local economies resonate as powerful notes in the melody of economic hope.

The transformation of healthcare systems becomes a key theme. The narratives of individuals working in healthcare, adapting to evolving medical landscapes, and contributing to public health initiatives become integral components of the evolving healthcare narrative of hope. The stories of healthcare professionals navigating challenges, implementing telemedicine solutions, and advocating for inclusive healthcare practices contribute to the symphony of hopeful change in the face of health uncertainties.

Cultural adaptations contribute to the vibrancy of the symphony. The narratives of artists exploring new mediums, cultural institutions embracing digital expressions, and communities reimagining traditional practices become integral components of the evolving cultural landscape of hope. The stories of resilience in the face of cultural challenges, the celebration of diverse expressions, and the commitment to preserving cultural heritage contribute to the symphony of cultural hope.

Global Interconnectedness: Harmony in Diversity

In the post-Omicron world, hope finds resonance in the harmonious notes of global interconnectedness. The narratives of individuals and nations collaborating, supporting one another, and recognizing shared destinies contribute to the evolving geopolitical landscape of hope. The stories of diplomatic dialogues, international collaborations, and a shared commitment to global well-being become integral components of the symphony of hope that transcends borders.

Global health initiatives become symbols of shared hope. The narratives of individuals and organizations working toward equitable vaccine distribution, supporting healthcare systems in need, and fostering global cooperation in public health contribute to the evolving global narrative of hope. The stories of nations coming together to address health challenges, share resources, and recognize the importance of global health security resonate as powerful notes in the symphony of global hope.

Environmental collaborations become essential threads in the tapestry of global hope. The narratives of nations working together to address climate change, protect biodiversity, and

promote sustainable practices contribute to the evolving environmental narrative of hope. The stories of international agreements, collaborative research, and a shared commitment to environmental stewardship resonate as harmonious notes in the symphony of global hope.

Educational partnerships become bridges of hope between nations. The narratives of collaborative educational initiatives, student exchanges, and cross-cultural learning experiences contribute to the evolving educational narrative of hope. The stories of nations supporting one another in educational endeavors, fostering understanding through academic exchanges, and recognizing the importance of global perspectives in education resonate as essential notes in the symphony of global hope.

Challenges and Opportunities in the Melody of Hope

Amidst the harmonious melody of hope, challenges and opportunities emerge as integral components of the symphony. The complexities of navigating personal, community, and global hope prompt ongoing reflections on the fragility and strength of the human spirit. The narratives of individuals grappling with uncertainties, addressing systemic challenges, and fostering environments that prioritize well-being become integral components of the evolving human story.

Economic disparities remain a challenge in the symphony of hope. The narratives of individuals navigating the impact of economic constraints, advocating for equitable opportunities, and fostering environments that prioritize economic inclusivity become reflections on the intersection of economic realities and hope. The understanding that hope must address issues of accessibility, representation, and economic well-being becomes a guiding principle in the exploration of economic challenges in the post-Omicron world.

Mental health disparities prompt ongoing considerations. The narratives of individuals navigating the complexities of mental health, addressing stigma, and fostering environments that prioritize emotional well-being become reflections on the challenges and opportunities inherent in the symphony of hope. The understanding that hope must extend to collective efforts, empathy, and a commitment to destigmatizing mental health becomes a central theme in the exploration of mental health challenges.

Social inequalities remain focal points in the evolving narrative of hope. The narratives of individuals challenging systemic injustices, advocating for social equity, and fostering environments that value diversity become reflections on the challenges and opportunities in the symphony of hope.

The understanding that hope requires intentional efforts to address systemic inequalities and create inclusive spaces becomes a guiding principle in the exploration of social challenges in the post-Omicron world.

The complexities of global interconnectedness prompt ongoing dialogues. The narratives of individuals navigating the challenges of geopolitical landscapes, contributing to global collaborations, and fostering environments that prioritize international cooperation become reflections on the opportunities and challenges inherent in the symphony of hope. The understanding that global hope requires diplomatic efforts, mutual support, and a recognition of shared vulnerabilities becomes a central theme in the exploration of global challenges in the post-Omicron era.

The Future of Hope: A Collective Symphony

As we navigate the melody of hope in the post-Omicron world, the future emerges as a collective symphony shaped by the stories, experiences, and aspirations of individuals and communities. From the triumphs of personal renewal to the harmonious collaboration of nations, each note in the symphony contributes to the rich narrative of hope.

The essence of hope lies in the recognition that challenges are inherent in the human experience, but so too is the capacity for renewal, resilience, and collective strength. The ongoing exploration of hope in the post-Omicron era becomes an invitation for individuals and nations to contribute their stories, experiences, and perspectives to the evolving human narrative. As communities engage in dialogues about the meaning of hope, the role of collective well-being, and the importance of fostering environments that nurture the human spirit, the symphony becomes a living testament to the beauty, strength, and transformative power of hope in the post-Omicron world.

Connections Rediscovered

In the post-Omicron landscape, a chapter unfolds that celebrates the rediscovery of connections—both personal and communal. As individuals and communities navigate the aftermath of the variant, the narratives of rediscovered connections become threads in the intricate tapestry of human experience. In this chapter, we explore the profound ways in which connections are revitalized, relationships are rekindled, and a sense of belonging is reaffirmed.

Personal Rediscovery: Navigating the Inner Landscape

At the heart of the chapter on rediscovery are the personal narratives that illuminate the inner landscapes of individuals. The journey of self-discovery, the reconnection with one's essence, and the embrace of authenticity become integral components of the evolving human story.

The rediscovery of personal identity becomes a transformative journey. Individuals share stories of self-reflection, embracing authenticity, and navigating the complexities of self-acceptance. The narratives of individuals exploring their passions, understanding their strengths, and embracing their unique identities contribute to the evolving tapestry of personal rediscovery.

Emotional landscapes are explored with newfound depth. Individuals share narratives of navigating complex emotions, fostering emotional resilience, and cultivating a deeper understanding of their own emotional well-being.

The stories of individuals engaging in practices that promote emotional health, seeking therapy, and creating environments that prioritize emotional well-being contribute to the evolving human narrative of personal rediscovery.

The pursuit of inner passions and creative expressions takes center stage. Individuals share stories of rediscovering hobbies, pursuing artistic endeavors, and embracing creativity as a form of self-expression. The narratives of individuals finding solace in creative pursuits, exploring new artistic mediums, and contributing to the cultural landscape with their expressions become integral components of the evolving tapestry of personal rediscovery.

Well-being practices and self-care rituals become essential components of personal rediscovery. Individuals share narratives of adopting healthy lifestyles, prioritizing mental health, and engaging in practices that contribute to overall well-being. The stories of individuals finding joy in self-care, exploring mindfulness practices, and fostering environments that prioritize holistic health contribute to the evolving human narrative of personal rediscovery.

Rekindling Relationships: The Dance of Interpersonal Connections

The chapter on connections rediscovered extends beyond personal narratives to encompass the dance of interpersonal relationships. The narratives of rekindled friendships, strengthened family bonds, and the revitalization of social connections become integral threads in the tapestry of communal rediscovery.

Friendships are reignited with the flame of shared experiences. Individuals share stories of reconnecting with long-lost friends, revitalizing friendships that stood the test of time, and creating spaces for shared joy. The narratives of individuals reaching out to old friends, fostering new connections, and recognizing the significance of friendship in their lives contribute to the evolving human story of interpersonal rediscovery.

Family bonds are strengthened through shared narratives and moments of togetherness. Individuals share stories of deepening connections with family members, finding new ways to appreciate familial ties, and navigating the complexities of family dynamics. The narratives of individuals fostering environments of love and support, celebrating family traditions, and recognizing the importance of familial connections in their lives contribute to the evolving tapestry of communal rediscovery.

Romantic relationships undergo a renewal of intimacy and understanding. Individuals share narratives of rekindling the flame in romantic partnerships, navigating challenges with open communication, and fostering environments of mutual growth. The stories of individuals investing in the emotional well-being of their relationships, embracing vulnerability, and finding joy in shared experiences become integral components of the evolving human narrative of interpersonal rediscovery.

Social connections in communities are revitalized. Individuals share stories of participating in communal activities, engaging in neighborhood initiatives, and contributing to the vibrancy of community life. The narratives of individuals recognizing the interconnectedness of their lives with those around them, fostering a sense of community belonging, and creating spaces for shared joy contribute to the evolving tapestry of communal rediscovery.

Cultural Reconnection: Embracing Heritage and Diversity

The chapter on connections rediscovered expands its focus to the cultural landscape, where individuals and communities reconnect with their heritage, celebrate diversity, and contribute to the richness of cultural expressions.

Individuals rediscover cultural roots and heritage. Narratives of individuals exploring their ancestral heritage, learning about cultural traditions, and embracing the richness of their cultural identity become integral components of the evolving tapestry of cultural rediscovery. The stories of individuals participating in cultural events, celebrating festivals, and passing down cultural practices to future generations contribute to the human narrative of cultural rediscovery.

Cultural diversity is celebrated with renewed enthusiasm. Narratives of individuals engaging with diverse cultural expressions, embracing global perspectives, and fostering environments that value inclusivity become integral components of the evolving cultural landscape of rediscovery. The stories of individuals contributing to cultural exchange, participating in cross-cultural dialogues, and recognizing the beauty of diversity contribute to the human narrative of cultural rediscovery.

Traditional practices are revitalized with contemporary relevance. Narratives of individuals infusing modern elements into traditional practices, reimagining cultural ceremonies, and adapting traditions to contemporary contexts become integral components of the evolving tapestry of cultural rediscovery. The stories of individuals finding meaning in cultural rituals, participating in cultural exchanges, and contributing to the preservation of cultural heritage contribute to the human narrative of cultural rediscovery.

Digital platforms play a central role in cultural reconnection. Narratives of individuals using technology to connect with global cultures, participate in virtual events, and foster digital collaborations become integral components of the evolving cultural landscape of rediscovery. The stories of individuals leveraging digital platforms to amplify cultural voices, connect with diverse communities, and create digital spaces that celebrate heritage contribute to the human narrative of cultural rediscovery.

Educational Reimagining: Nurturing Curiosity and Lifelong Learning

The chapter on connections rediscovered explores the educational landscape, where individuals and communities reimagine learning, nurture curiosity, and contribute to the lifelong pursuit of knowledge.

Lifelong learning becomes a cornerstone of personal and communal growth. Narratives of individuals engaging in continuous learning, pursuing new skills, and embracing educational opportunities throughout their lives become integral components of the evolving educational narrative of rediscovery. The stories of individuals participating in online courses, attending workshops, and recognizing the transformative power of education contribute to the human narrative of educational rediscovery.

Educational institutions foster environments of curiosity and exploration. Narratives of schools providing innovative learning experiences, educators inspiring curiosity in students, and educational institutions becoming hubs for intellectual growth become integral components of the evolving tapestry of educational rediscovery. The stories of individuals benefiting from inclusive curricula, engaging in hands-on learning experiences, and recognizing the value of curiosity in education contribute to the human narrative of educational rediscovery.

Communities become centers for knowledge exchange and collaborative learning. Narratives of individuals participating in community-based educational initiatives, attending local workshops, and contributing to the collective pursuit of knowledge become integral components of the evolving educational landscape of rediscovery. The stories of individuals recognizing the importance of community-driven learning, fostering spaces for intellectual exchange, and contributing to the educational well-being of their communities contribute to the human narrative of educational rediscovery.

Technology transforms the educational landscape. Narratives of individuals leveraging digital platforms for learning, participating in online educational communities, and embracing technology as a tool for educational exploration become integral components of the evolving educational narrative of rediscovery. The stories of individuals benefiting from accessible educational resources, engaging in virtual classrooms, and recognizing the potential of technology to democratize education contribute to the human narrative of educational rediscovery.

Challenges and Opportunities in the Rediscovery of Connections

Within the tapestry of rediscovered connections, challenges and opportunities emerge

as integral components. The complexities of navigating personal, communal, and cultural rediscovery prompt ongoing reflections on the fragility and resilience of human connections. The narratives of individuals grappling with uncertainties, addressing systemic challenges, and fostering environments that prioritize connection become integral components of the evolving human story.

The challenge of navigating changing relationships prompts reflections. Narratives of individuals grappling with shifts in personal connections, redefining boundaries in relationships, and addressing the complexities of evolving social dynamics become reflections on the challenges and opportunities inherent in the rediscovery of connections. The understanding that connection requires intentional efforts, open communication, and a commitment to mutual growth becomes a guiding principle in the exploration of relational challenges in the post-Omicron world.

The complexity of embracing cultural diversity prompts ongoing dialogues. Narratives of individuals navigating cultural exchanges, challenging stereotypes, and fostering environments that celebrate diversity become reflections on the challenges and opportunities in the rediscovery of connections. The understanding that connection requires empathy, cultural understanding, and a recognition of shared humanity becomes a central theme in the exploration of cultural challenges in the post-Omicron era.

The challenge of reimagining education prompts reflections on the future of learning. Narratives of individuals adapting to new educational landscapes, embracing digital learning platforms, and contributing to the evolution of educational paradigms become reflections on the challenges and opportunities in the rediscovery of connections. The understanding that connection requires inclusive educational practices, a commitment to lifelong learning, and a recognition of the transformative power of knowledge becomes a guiding principle in the exploration of educational challenges in the post-Omicron world.

The complexity of fostering communal connections prompts ongoing considerations. Narratives of individuals navigating community dynamics, participating in local initiatives, and contributing to the well-being of their communities become reflections on the challenges and opportunities in the rediscovery of connections. The understanding that connection requires collective efforts, a commitment to community well-being, and a recognition of the interconnectedness of individual and communal lives becomes a central theme in the exploration of communal challenges in the post-Omicron era.

The Future of Rediscovered Connections: A Tapestry of Human Experience

As we navigate the tapestry of rediscovered connections in the post-Omicron world, the future emerges as a collective work of art shaped by the stories, experiences, and aspirations of individuals and communities. From the rekindling of personal relationships to the celebration of cultural diversity, each thread in the tapestry contributes to the rich narrative of human connection.

The essence of connection lies in the recognition that relationships are dynamic, cultures are ever-evolving, and education is a lifelong journey. The ongoing exploration of rediscovered connections becomes an invitation for individuals and communities to contribute their stories, experiences, and perspectives to the evolving human narrative. As we engage in dialogues about the meaning of connection, the role of collective well-being, and the importance of fostering environments that nurture human connections, the tapestry becomes a living testament to the beauty, resilience, and transformative power of rediscovered connections in the post-Omicron world.

Embracing Tomorrow

In the wake of the Omicron variant, a chapter unfolds—one that beckons individuals and communities to embrace tomorrow with open hearts and a collective spirit. As the echoes of the variant gradually fade, the narratives of resilience, rediscovery, and hope converge into a symphony of possibilities. In this chapter, we explore the multifaceted dimensions of embracing tomorrow, delving into the stories of adaptation, renewal, and the indomitable human spirit that paves the way for a brighter future.

Adapting to the Evolving Landscape: The Dance of Flexibility

At the core of the chapter on embracing tomorrow are the personal narratives that illuminate the journey of adaptation. Individuals share stories of navigating the uncertainties of the post-Omicron world, embracing change, and discovering the resilience inherent in adaptability.

The journey of professional adaptation becomes a testament to human ingenuity. Individuals share narratives of pivoting careers, embracing remote work, and finding innovative solutions to economic challenges. The stories of individuals navigating the complexities of a changing job market, upskilling for new opportunities, and contributing to the evolving professional landscape become integral components of the evolving human narrative of adaptation.

Personal lives undergo transformations with a spirit of flexibility. Individuals share stories of adjusting to new routines, finding joy in simplicity, and fostering environments that prioritize well-being. The narratives of individuals navigating the complexities of family dynamics, embracing change in personal relationships, and recognizing the importance of emotional well-being contribute to the evolving tapestry of human adaptation.

Educational landscapes witness innovative adaptations. Individuals share narratives of students and educators navigating hybrid learning environments, embracing digital tools, and contributing to the evolving educational narrative. The stories of individuals participating in online courses, engaging in virtual classrooms, and recognizing the potential of technology to democratize education contribute to the evolving human narrative of adaptation in the educational sphere.

The embrace of technological advancements becomes a hallmark of adaptation. Individuals share stories of leveraging digital platforms for communication, connection, and collaboration. The narratives of individuals contributing to the digital landscape, engaging in virtual communities, and recognizing the transformative power of technology in daily life become integral components of the evolving human story of adaptation.

Renewing Cultural Expressions: The Vibrancy of Shared Creativity

The chapter on embracing tomorrow extends its focus to the cultural landscape, where individuals and communities renew expressions of creativity, celebrate diversity, and contribute to the richness of cultural tapestries.

Artistic expressions become vibrant notes in the symphony of cultural renewal. Individuals share narratives of artists exploring new mediums, cultural institutions embracing digital expressions, and communities reimagining traditional practices. The stories of resilience in the face of cultural challenges, the celebration of diverse expressions, and the commitment to preserving cultural heritage contribute to the evolving cultural landscape of renewal.

Cultural diversity is celebrated with renewed enthusiasm. Narratives of individuals engaging with diverse cultural expressions, embracing global perspectives, and fostering environments that value inclusivity become integral components of the evolving cultural landscape of renewal. The stories of individuals contributing to cultural exchange, participating in cross-cultural dialogues, and recognizing the beauty of diversity contribute to the human narrative of cultural renewal.

Traditional practices are revitalized with contemporary relevance. Narratives of individuals infusing modern elements into traditional practices, reimagining cultural ceremonies, and adapting traditions to contemporary contexts become integral components of the evolving tapestry of cultural renewal. The stories of individuals finding meaning in cultural rituals, participating in cultural exchanges, and contributing to the preservation of cultural heritage contribute to the human narrative of cultural renewal.

Digital platforms play a central role in cultural renewal. Narratives of individuals using technology to connect with global cultures, participate in virtual events, and foster digital collaborations become integral components of the evolving cultural landscape of renewal. The stories of individuals leveraging digital platforms to amplify cultural voices, connect with diverse communities, and create digital spaces that celebrate heritage contribute to the human narrative of cultural renewal.

Community Collaborations: The Strength of Collective Endeavors

The chapter on embracing tomorrow explores the communal landscape, where individuals and communities collaborate, support one another, and contribute to the well-being of collective spaces.

Community-led initiatives become beacons of collective strength. Individuals share stories of coming together to address local challenges, foster inclusivity, and create spaces for collective well-being. The narratives of individuals supporting one another, grassroots organizations leading change, and communities becoming hubs for resilience resonate as powerful notes in the symphony of communal renewal.

Cultural celebrations and expressions mark a chapter of communal renewal. Communities share stories of reviving traditional practices, hosting festivals, and embracing the vibrancy of cultural diversity. The narratives of individuals participating in cultural events, supporting local artists, and fostering environments that celebrate heritage contribute to the evolving cultural landscape of communal renewal.

Environmental stewardship becomes a shared commitment within communities. Narratives of individuals and groups advocating for sustainable practices, engaging in conservation efforts, and prioritizing environmental well-being contribute to the evolving environmental narrative of communal renewal. The stories of communities fostering green initiatives, implementing eco-friendly practices, and raising awareness about the interconnectedness of human and environmental health resonate as essential notes in the symphony of communal renewal.

Educational initiatives within communities become centers for collective growth. Narratives of individuals participating in community-based educational initiatives, attending local workshops, and contributing to the collective pursuit of knowledge become integral components of the evolving educational landscape of communal renewal. The stories of individuals recognizing the importance of community-driven learning, fostering spaces for intellectual exchange, and contributing to the educational well-being of their communities contribute to the human narrative of communal renewal.

Global Interconnectedness: Navigating Tomorrow Together

In the post-Omicron world, the theme of global interconnectedness becomes even more pronounced. The narratives of individuals and nations collaborating, supporting one another, and recognizing shared destinies contribute to the evolving geopolitical landscape of global renewal.

Global health initiatives become symbols of shared commitment. Narratives of individuals and organizations working toward equitable vaccine distribution, supporting healthcare systems in need, and fostering global cooperation in public health contribute to the evolving global narrative of renewal. The stories of nations coming together to address health challenges, share resources, and recognize the importance of global health security resonate as powerful notes in the symphony of global renewal.

Environmental collaborations become essential threads in the tapestry of global renewal. Narratives of nations working together to address climate change, protect biodiversity, and promote sustainable practices contribute to the evolving environmental narrative of global renewal. The stories of international agreements, collaborative research, and a shared commitment to environmental stewardship resonate as harmonious notes in the symphony of global renewal.

Educational partnerships become bridges of hope between nations. Narratives of collaborative educational initiatives, student exchanges, and cross-cultural learning experiences contribute to the evolving educational narrative of global renewal. The stories of nations supporting one another in educational endeavors, fostering understanding through academic exchanges, and recognizing the importance of global perspectives in education resonate as essential notes in the symphony of global renewal.

Challenges and Opportunities in Embracing Tomorrow

Within the symphony of embracing tomorrow, challenges and opportunities emerge as integral components. The complexities of navigating personal, communal, and global renewal prompt ongoing reflections on the fragility and strength of human endeavors. The narratives of individuals grappling with uncertainties, addressing systemic challenges, and fostering environments that prioritize collective well-being become integral components of the evolving human story.

Economic disparities remain a challenge in the symphony of renewal. Narratives of individuals navigating the impact of economic constraints, advocating for equitable opportunities, and fostering environments that prioritize economic inclusivity become reflections on the intersection of economic realities and renewal. The understanding that renewal

must address issues of accessibility, representation, and economic well-being becomes a guiding principle in the exploration of economic challenges in the post-Omicron world.

Mental health disparities prompt ongoing considerations. Narratives of individuals navigating the complexities of mental health, addressing stigma, and fostering environments that prioritize emotional well-being become reflections on the challenges and opportunities inherent in the symphony of renewal. The understanding that renewal must extend to collective efforts, empathy, and a commitment to destigmatizing mental health becomes a central theme in the exploration of mental health challenges.

Social inequalities remain focal points in the evolving narrative of renewal. Narratives of individuals challenging systemic injustices, advocating for social equity, and fostering environments that value diversity become reflections on the challenges and opportunities in the symphony of renewal. The understanding that renewal requires intentional efforts to address systemic inequalities and create inclusive spaces becomes a guiding principle in the exploration of social challenges in the post-Omicron world.

The complexities of global interconnectedness prompt ongoing dialogues. Narratives of individuals navigating the challenges of geopolitical landscapes, contributing to global collaborations, and fostering environments that prioritize international cooperation become reflections on the opportunities and challenges inherent in the symphony of renewal. The understanding that global renewal requires diplomatic efforts, mutual support, and a recognition of shared vulnerabilities becomes a central theme in the exploration of global challenges in the post-Omicron era.

The Future of Embracing Tomorrow: A Collective Symphony of Renewal

As we navigate the symphony of embracing tomorrow in the post-Omicron world, the future emerges as a collective symphony shaped by the stories, experiences, and aspirations of individuals and communities. From the triumphs of personal adaptation to the celebration of cultural diversity, each note in the symphony contributes to the rich narrative of human renewal.

The essence of renewal lies in the recognition that challenges are inherent in the human experience, but so too is the capacity for adaptation, resilience, and collective strength. The ongoing exploration of renewal in the post-Omicron era becomes an invitation for individuals and nations to contribute their stories, experiences, and perspectives to the evolving human narrative. As communities engage in dialogues about the meaning of renewal, the role of collective well-being, and the importance of fostering environments that nurture human endeavors, the symphony becomes a living testament to the beauty, strength, and transformative power of embracing tomorrow in the post-Omicron world.

www.ingramcontent.com/pod-product-compliance
Lightning Source LLC
LaVergne TN
LVHW051054180726
843512LV00019B/1465